Jewish Perspectives
on Theology
and the Human Experience
of Disability

Jewish Perspectives on Theology and the Human Experience of Disability has been co-published simultaneously as *Journal of Religion, Disability & Health*, Volume 10, Numbers 3/4 2006.

Monographic Separates from the *Journal of Religion, Disability & Health*™

For additional information on these and other Haworth Press titles, including descriptions, tables of contents, reviews, and prices, use the QuickSearch catalog at http://www.HaworthPress.com.

Jewish Perspectives on Theology and the Human Experience of Disability, edited by Rabbi Judith Z. Abrams, PhD, and William C. Gaventa, MDiv (Vol. 10, No. 3/4, 2006). *"Offers an inclusive kaleidoscopic view of Judaism and how Judaism approaches disability. Each sensitive contribution adds depth and perspective to the moral imperatives confronting Jewish law, individuals, families, communities and humanity. Read in parts or as a whole, this work is an instrumental text for study, exploration and great comfort." (Rabbi Michal Hyman, MA, Chaplain, UCLA Medical Center)*

Disability Advocacy Among Religious Organizations: Histories and Reflections, edited by Albert A. Herzog, Jr., PhD, MDiv, MA (Vol. 10, No. 1/2, 2006). *Insightful exploration of the histories of disability advocacy within numerous religious organizations since 1950.*

End-of-Life Care: Bridging Disability and Aging with Person-Centered Care, edited by Rev. William C. Gaventa, MDiv, and David L. Coulter, MD (Vol. 9, No. 2, 2005). *A probing set of examinations into disability, Alzheimer's, and end-of-life debates, using a pair of cogent arguments as a starting point, followed by carefully considered responses from other experts.*

Critical Reflections on Stanley Hauerwas' Theology of Disability: Disabling Society, Enabling Theology, edited by John Swinton, PhD (Vol. 8, No. 3/4, 2004). *"AN EXCELLENT AND LONG-NEEDED RESOURCE. . . . This work will not only continue the ongoing discussion among those specializing in the theology of disability in general and disability related to intellectual development in particular, but will also serve to bring disability into the mainline of contemporary theological discussion." (Kerry H. Wynn, PhD, Director, Learning Enrichment Center, Southeast Missouri State University)*

Voices in Disability and Spirituality from the Land Down Under: From Outback to Outfront, edited by Rev. Dr. Christopher Newell, PhD, and Rev. Andy Calder (Vol. 8, No. 1/2, 2004). *"In recent years disability theology has emerged alongside Black theology and womens' theology as a new genre seeking to express the concerns of people whose experience has often been marginalized. This collection is A SIGNIFICANT AUSTRALIAN CONTRIBUTION TO THIS GROWING LITERATURE. The early explorers named Australia 'the south land of the Holy Spirit.' (John M. Hull, PhD, Hon DTheol, Professor Emeritus of Religious Education, University of Birmingham, England; Author of* On Sight and Insight *and* In the Beginning There Was Darkness).*

Graduate Theological Education and the Human Experience of Disability, edited by Robert C. Anderson (Vol. 7, No. 3, 2003). *"A comprehensive overview of theological education and disability. . . . Concise and well written. . . . Offers rich theological insights and abundant practical advice. I strongly recommend this volume as a key introduction to this important emerging topic in theological education." (Rev. John W. Crossin, PhD, OSFS, Executive Director, Washington Theological Consortium)*

The Pastoral Voice of Robert Perske, edited by William C. Gaventa, Jr., MDiv, and David L. Coulter, MD (Vol. 7, No. 1/2, 2003). *"Must reading for seminary students and clinical program directors. Pastors, providers, and parents concerned with persons suffering from cognitive, intellectual, and developmental disabilities will find these vigorous testimonies readable, timely, fresh, and inspiring despite having been written more than 30 years ago." (Barbara J. Lampe, JD, Executive Director, National Apostolate for Inclusion Ministry)*

Jewish Perspectives on Theology and the Human Experience of Disability

Rabbi Judith Z. Abrams, PhD
William C. Gaventa, MDiv
Editors

Jewish Perspectives on Theology and the Human Experience of Disability has been co-published simultaneously as *Journal of Religion, Disability & Health*, Volume 10, Numbers 3/4 2006.

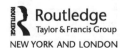

Routledge
Taylor & Francis Group
NEW YORK AND LONDON

Published by

The Haworth Pastoral Press®, 10 Alice Street, Binghamton, NY 13904-1580 USA

The Haworth Pastoral Press® is an imprint of The Haworth Press, Inc., 10 Alice Street, Binghamton, NY 13904-1580 USA.

Jewish Perspectives on Theology and the Human Experience of Disability has been co-published simultaneously as *Journal of Religion, Disability & Health*, Volume 10, Numbers 3/4 2006.

Library of Congress Cataloging-in-Publication Data

Jewish perspectives on theology and the human experience of disability /Judith Z. Abrams, and William C. Gaventa, editors.
    p. cm.
    Co-published simultaneously as Journal of religion, disability & health, v. 10, no. 3-4, 2006.
    Includes bibliographical references and index.
    ISBN-13: 978-0-7890-3444-1 (hard cover : alk. paper)
    ISBN-10: 0-7890-3444-1 (hard cover : alk. paper)
    ISBN-13: 978-0-7890-3445-8 (soft cover : alk. paper)
    ISBN-10: 0-7890-3445-X (soft cover : alk. paper)
    1. People with disabilities–Religious aspects–Judaism. I. Abrams, Judith Z. II. Gaventa, William C. III. Journal of religion, disability & health.
BM540.H35J49 2006
296.3087–dc22
                                        2006015776

Jewish Perspectives on Theology and the Human Experience of Disability

CONTENTS

CONCLUDING CONTEMPLATION

BOOK REVIEWS

ABOUT THE EDITORS

Rabbi Judith Z. Abrams, PhD, is Founder and Director of Maqom: A School for Adult Talmud Study in Houston, Texas. She was ordained at Hebrew Union College in 1985 and earned her PhD in Rabbinic Literature from the Baltimore Hebrew University in 1993. Rabbi Abrams received the Covenant Award in 1999, presented each year by the Covenant Foundation to outstanding Jewish educators in North America. Her latest book, *Torah and Company* (Ben Yahuda Press), is her 18th.

William C. Gaventa, MDiv, is Associate Professor in the Department of Pediatrics at the Robert Wood Johnson Medical School and Director of Community and Congregational Supports at the Elizabeth M. Boggs Center of Developmental Disabilities in New Brunswick, New Jersey. He also coordinates a training and technical assistance team for New Jersey Self Determination Initiative, which now supports more than 300 individuals and their families. In 2006, he received the New Jersey Coalition for Inclusive Ministries/Open R.O.A.D. Award in recognition of his contributions and commitment to people with disabilities.

Mr. Gaventa also serves as coordinator of Family Support for the Georgia Developmental Disabilities Council, Chaplain and Coordinator of Religious Services for the Monroe Developmental Center, and Executive Secretary for the Religion Division of the AAMR since 1985. He served on the Board of Directors of the AAMR, 2002-2005. He is co-editor of *The Theological Voice of Wolf Wolfensberger*; *Spirituality and Intellectual Disability: International Perspectives on the Effect of Culture and Religion on Healing Body, Mind, and Soul*; and *The Pastoral Voice of Robert Perske*, all from Haworth Press.

Foreword

This collection of articles and authors represents in many ways the best of what this series of volumes hope to embody. The authors and perspectives come from across the broad dimensions of Judaism, from a number of roles (theologian, rabbis, parents, lawyers, and persons with disabilities), and from across the world: Israel, the United States, the United Kingdom, and Australia. They include theology, scripture, history, ethics, practical theology, religious education, and personal experience; many voices, from many places, struggling within a major faith tradition to understand and apply the lessons, wisdom and revelation of history to the lived experience and questions of the present.

It has been my honor and privilege at a number of times in my interfaith work with people with disabilities, their families, and their faith communities to be part of Jewish services, programs and experiences. This ex-Baptist missionary kid can honestly say that some of the most sacred moments in my own faith journey have come through those experiences. Accompanying a group of adults from a developmental center to their first Rosh Hashanah service in years, seeing them along with a young refugee from Russia gather around the rabbi and the Torah after the service, being given a prayer shawl by a Jewish psychologist in Melbourne in October, 2001 with the mission of bringing it back to the States to find a young boy whose father had been killed in 9/11, sharing in Passover seders, being part of a bar mitzvah service done by local synagogues for adults from a nearby institution who had never had the opportunity, learning to sing some of the songs, working with Ilana Trachtman as she produces *Praying with Lior*. . . the list goes on and on.

[Haworth co-indexing entry note]: "Foreword." Gaventa, William C. Co-published simultaneously in *Journal of Religion, Disability & Health* (The Haworth Pastoral Press, an imprint of The Haworth Press, Inc.) Vol. 10, No. 3/4, 2006, pp. xxi-xxiii; and: *Jewish Perspectives on Theology and the Human Experience of Disability* (ed: Rabbi Judith Z. Abrams, and William C. Gaventa) The Haworth Pastoral Press, an imprint of The Haworth Press, Inc., 2006, pp. xv-xvii. Single or multiple copies of this article are available for a fee from The Haworth Document Delivery Service [1-800-HAWORTH, 9:00 a.m. - 5:00 p.m. (EST). E-mail address: docdelivery@haworthpress.com].

Now I can add to that list the experience of reading these pieces and shaping them into a collection with Rabbi Abrams. I inherited the task from Robert Anderson who first received some of these articles when his call for papers for a volume on theological education (VII. 2) led to a number of Jewish submissions, and a decision to try to focus a volume on that tradition. Bob and I enlisted Rabbi Abrams, for it would have been beyond chutzpah for two Christians to edit a volume of pieces written by, and primarily for, the Jewish community. The demands of Bob Anderson's own graduate program led to my taking over his role, and now, at long last, our completion of this collection with the help of Rabbi Judith Abrams, the author of one of the two primary books about Judaism and disability which have been published in the last decade. We are very grateful for her guidance and assistance.

But if you think this is just a collection for Jewish readers, you would be very wrong. Read the first two articles by Rabbi Artson and Wallace Greene. If you are not hooked, I will be surprised. There is a richness of story, a depth of commitment and scholarship, and a willingness to wrestle with understandings of G-d, tradition, and experience that comes through over and over again. A careful reading will shatter stereotypes of Judaism and common interpretations of scripture. For example, the Leviticus passages have long been cited as evidence of discrimination by religious communities and traditions. But read more deeply and carefully, and re-applied, several authors help us see those texts anew. The story and tradition of Rabbi Pereidah, with his practice of giving a slow child at least 400 chances, simply humbles us in an age when we are tempted to blame slow learning on a child because of his or her disability. In that story, you can almost hear an ancestor of Marc Gold, one of the first champions of supported employment, challenging us. Marc Gold used to say that when we think a person with an intellectual disability cannot learn, it says more about our ability to teach than it does about his or her capacity to learn.

We are indeed grateful to the authors for their work, to organizations that originally published some of these pieces for permission to republish, and for everyone's capacity to demonstrate a time-honored characteristic of faith, i.e., patience, through the time it took to get this collection to print. There are exciting and new forms of telling new Jewish stories that are coming just over the horizon, as Ilana Trachtman finishes her editing of the documentary on Lior, a young man with Down Syndrome and his journey toward his bar mitzvah (*www.prayingwithlior.com*) and groups like the Council For Jews With Special Needs in Phoenix and the Jewish Community Inclusion Program for People with Disabilities in Minneapolis St. Paul work hard on communities of inclusion at every level. Our hope is that this collection becomes a valuable tool in those and other initiatives within Jewish traditions while it also serves as a light for others who share some of the same scriptures and others still who share the call to revisit sacred stories, texts, and traditions to find, once again, new ways of using them to understand and inform current experience.

William C. Gaventa, MDiv
Co-Editor
Journal of Religion, Disability & Health

Introduction

Rabbi Judith Z. Abrams, PhD

A recognition of disabilities and their role in Jewish life is evident from our earliest to our most recent sources. From the Torah to modern writing, Judaism takes account of persons with disabilities and their role in the community. The broad sweep of the articles in this volume supports this assertion by providing ample evidence of these claims.

We begin and end with the contemplations about disabilities by Bradley Shavit Artson. He notes that, "history won't remove the problem for most of us" when contemplating ancient texts and their apparent attitudes toward disabilities. Rather, he suggests, it is the immediate experience and acceptance of persons with disabilities that should inform tradition.

The three main movements of Judaism–Orthodox, Conservative and Reform–approach persons with disabilities in their own distinctive ways. Wallace Greene's piece, "Jewish Theological Approaches to the Human Experience of Disability" reflects an Orthodox stance. In his view, "We need to move beyond seeing people with disabilities as needy and toward a view that all people have needs. This model stresses interdependency as a central characteristic of life and society."

The Conservative movement's Committee on Jewish Law and Standards decides that movement's stance on important issues. Daniel S. Nevin's article is a record of the Committee's deliberation regarding

Rabbi Judith Z. Abrams, PhD, is affiliated with Maqom: A School for Adult Talmud Study, P.O. B. 31900-323, Houston, TX 77231 (E-mail: maqom@compassnet.com).

[Haworth co-indexing entry note]: "Introduction." Abrams, Rabbi Judith Z. Co-published simultaneously in *Journal of Religion, Disability & Health* (The Haworth Pastoral Press, an imprint of The Haworth Press, Inc.) Vol. 10, No. 3/4, 2006, pp. 1-3; and: *Jewish Perspectives on Theology and the Human Experience of Disability* (ed: Rabbi Judith Z. Abrams, and William C. Gaventa) The Haworth Pastoral Press, an imprint of The Haworth Press, Inc., 2006, pp. 1-3. Single or multiple copies of this article are available for a fee from The Haworth Document Delivery Service [1-800-HAWORTH, 9:00 a.m. - 5:00 p.m. (EST). E-mail address: docdelivery@haworthpress.com].

Available online at http://jrdh.haworthpress.com
doi:10.1300/J095v10n03_01

how a blind person may participate in the Torah service. After an exhaustive examination of the sources which apply to this topic, the conclusion that the blind may participate in the Torah service in limited ways reflects both the decision-making process of that movement as well as its general stance, finding a way to both hold fast to the past while adapting to the present.

The Reform movement's rabbinic decision-making body, the Central Conference of American Rabbis' Responsa Committee, has been asked many questions which deal with disabilities over the years. Walter Jacob, who presided over the Committee for many years, was able to address these issues not only from a scholarly point of view but from a personal one as well. In his decision about a parent's obligation to visit a profoundly retarded child, he writes, "As I view this problem through my personal experience with a severely handicapped daughter . . . it is clear that unless ongoing relationships of some kind are established with such a handicapped child, the parents and other children will always feel guilty." The selection of other responsa presented here deal with handicapped access to a synagogue, divorce of an incapacitated spouse, and the ability of a blind person to serve as a witness (which allows a partial contrast between the Conservative and Reform stances regarding persons with disabilities).

In the next section, we have two articles which address the issue of disabilities from a more theoretical and scholarly framework. My own article seeks to dispel the erroneous notion that the requirements for priestly perfection found in the Torah apply to all Israelites. This misconception has led to the notion that the Torah limits disabled Israelites' participation in Jewish life. Why must the priests be physically perfect? "Because of the danger which was liable to befall those who approached this holy area (i.e., the Tabernacle) improperly." A blemishless body was needed as a sort of protective suit if a person were to come into contact with God's lethal presence.

Bonnie Gracer examines rabbinic attitudes toward persons with disabilities in her exploration of deafness in the *Mishnah*. She finds that, "In contrast to the evidence of infanticide as a response to disability in ancient Greece and Rome, the *Mishnah* records no debates on whether people with disabilities should be allowed to live; infanticide is never even raised as a possibility. Quite the contrary–the rabbis cherish life and see human variety as evidence of God's greatness."

In our final major section, we examine Judaism's theology regarding persons with disabilities and how that disability is put into action. Melinda Jones' article not only outlines a theology of inclusiveness and empowerment but advocates change when current religious practice differs from this theology: "My hope would be that there would be a re-examination of Jewish law to adjust it to modern times." Such a theology offers "not only hope but also help to people with disabilities."

The rest of the articles in this section demonstrate how this theology is being put into action today. The next three articles are descriptions of actual programs that addressed the issue of persons with disabilities in Jewish communal life today. Becca Hornstein's description of screening for Jewish genetic diseases, Eve Hersov's thorough and meaningful report on Jewish identity and disabled persons in Britain and the summary of the Minneapolis Jewish Community's Inclusion Program for People with Disabilities demonstrate that the articles in this volume are far from theoretical: they are becoming reality in Jewish life. Kandel et al. examine the issue of how marriage and parenthood among those with mental disabilities functions in today's world. Deena R. Zimmerman's article, "The Participation of Disabled Women in the Rules of *Niddah*" explores how disabled women in Israel can participate in the rite of the ritual bath, noting that "accommodations have to be made for the inclusion of the disabled in this part of religious practice." Robert Brown, writing from both a textual and a personal point of view, shows how modern technologies are making it possible for more persons with disabilities to participate in Talmud study, one of the core experiences of Jewish life.

While this volume offers a great deal of material it is by no means an exhaustive examination of the topic. In particular, for those wishing to create a course with this as a reader, I suggest including pages 234-237 of John Hockenberry's *Moving Violations: A Memoir* (Hyperion, 1995). Hockenberry is a paraplegic who lived in Israel and other countries in the Middle East as a reporter. His insights give the reader a bird's eye view of the day-to-day life of a person with disabilities in modern Israel. More insights about the role of disabilities in Israeli life–particularly disabilities and their role in the Israeli military experience–would have been welcome. This is a fruitful area for further research and documentation.

The study of disabilities, and the study of Judaism and disabilities is swelling with a rising tide of interest as people are becoming aware that very few people will live a life without being touched by this issue, either personally or by having a relative or friend with disabilities. This volume represents the vanguard of scholarship on this topic which will doubtless grow as time passes.

OPENING CONTEMPLATION

'Im ani kan, hakol kan
If I Am Here, All Is Here:
A Contemplation
on "Defects" and "Wholeness"

Rabbi Bradley Shavit Artson, MA

SUMMARY. The author provides an understanding that the community is incomplete without the presence and participation of people with disabilities. "The Torah was not given to angels. We are all of us blemished; human wholeness does not come from some elusive perfection, but rather from the radical act of taking hold of our imperfections and offering even them." The Torah reminds us of an insistence on a community that includes

Rabbi Bradley Shavit Artson is Dean, Ziegler School of Rabbinic Studies, and Vice-President, University of Judaism. Rabbi Artson is author of *The Bedside Torah* (McGraw-Hill). He writes a free weekly email Torah commentary, "Today's Torah." Address correspondence to: (E-mail: bartson@uj.edu).

[Haworth co-indexing entry note]: " '*Im ani kan, hakol kan* If I Am Here, All is Here: A Contemplation on 'Defects' and 'Wholeness'." Artson, Rabbi Bradley Shavit. Co-published simultaneously in *Journal of Religion, Disability & Health* (The Haworth Pastoral Press, an imprint of The Haworth Press, Inc.) Vol. 10, No. 3/4, 2006, pp. 5-8; and: *Jewish Perspectives on Theology and the Human Experience of Disability* (ed: Rabbi Judith Z. Abrams, and William C. Gaventa) The Haworth Pastoral Press, an imprint of The Haworth Press, Inc., 2006, pp. 5-8. Single or multiple copies of this article are available for a fee from The Haworth Document Delivery Service [1-800-HAWORTH, 9:00 a.m. - 5:00 p.m. (EST). E-mail address: docdelivery@haworthpress.com].

Available online at http://jrdh.haworthpress.com
© 2006 by The Haworth Press, Inc. All rights reserved.
doi:10.1300/J095v10n03_02

all of its members–that makes none of them invisible, that asks none to step outside. doi:10.1300/J095v10n03_02 *[Article copies available for a fee from The Haworth Document Delivery Service: 1-800-HAWORTH. E-mail address: <docdelivery@haworthpress.com> Website: <http://www.HaworthPress.com>*

KEYWORDS. Disability, Leviticus, blemish, wholeness, Torah

How do we measure human worth? What constitutes wholeness or greatness? And, by way of contrast, what constitutes a defect, an imperfection that renders another person less than complete? These questions intrude when we consider the lives of people with disabilities. They intrude as well when we peer into the depths of our own hearts and face our inner selves in the naked light of honesty. Disability disrupts the images of perfection that surround us and cry out: are we really good enough to do the tasks at hand? Are we pure enough? Are we holy enough? Has the Torah gone through our beings to transform us into someone sufficiently decent? Won't our shortcomings become immediately apparent, and immediately visible?

I'd like to create room to rethink the way we conceive our challenges, our imperfections, our embodiment, through the light of Torah. In addressing who is permitted to bring a sacrifice in the Holy Temple in Jerusalem, the Torah imposes the following restriction: *Ish mizeracha l'dorotam asher yiheyeh bo mum, lo yikra lehakriv lechem l'elohav; ki chol ish asher bo mum lo yikrav*–"No one of your offspring throughout the ages who has a defect–a *mum*–shall be qualified to offer food to God; no one who has a *mum*–a defect–shall be qualified" (Leviticus 21:17).

I have been schooled in the historical method of religious study. My first defense against troubling verses in the Torah is to quarantine them securely behind a historical context, so let us begin our contemplation using that approach. The Kohen in the Temple is understood to be a symbol of perfection. Because the Temple ritual is physical, the Kohen's perfection must also be physical. And that perfection is understood by the biblical text as *shleimut*–as wholeness. Therefore, the Kohen can't be missing any body part, because he has to literally embody that wholeness in the presence of God. Indeed, as the Torah goes on to state, *ach el ha-parochet lo yavo'u, v'el ha-mizbeach lo yigash, ki mum bo*–"One who has a defect shall not enter behind the curtain, nor come near the altar" (Leviticus 21:23).

But history won't remove the problem for most of us. Are we then saying that we can't draw near to God, we cannot serve on behalf of the community, if we have a *mum*, a defect? Is there anyone among us who is perfect? Is there anyone–anywhere–who doesn't, in fact, manifest not one *mum* but many? Is it possible that only those who are perfect are capable of serving God and of serving each other? Certainly, on a literal level, this has not been true in Jewish life. Our father Jacob "limped" his way into greatness. Moses spoke what are surely history's greatest orations with a speech impediment. The Talmud is filled with great figures–Nahum ish Gamzo, Rav Sheshet, and others–who, with their physical blemishes, perhaps because of them, went on to attain spiritual greatness. And then, theologically, certain it is that God is the only one who is perfect. Can it be, then, that only God can serve?

The Torah raises a question in the book of *Devarim. Shichet lo? Lo! banav mumam*–"Is corruption then God's? No, God's children are the ones who are blemished" (Deuteronomy 32:5). Rabbinic genius turns the verse around: "*Af al pi shehem m'laim mumim, kruim banim*–even though they are full of imperfections, they are still God's children" (*Sifri Devarim*, Parashat Ha'azinu, Piska 3).

We are–all of us–God's children, blemishes, defects, imperfections and all, and we cannot afford to allow human shortcomings or disabilities to prevent us from taking the responsibility that is ours to do what good we can, to glorify Torah and to testify to God's sovereignty as we might. So I'd like to try to offer a different percolation of that initial verse in *Parashat Emor*. A *mum* is that lack which makes us feel incomplete. It is the part of some imaginary whole. I would like to propose, then, that wholeness does not mean physical perfection. Indeed, *shleimut* is not perfection of any kind. *Shleimut* means serving God with all our being, with the entirety of who we are, with leaving no part of ourselves outside of the divine service–*bechol levav'cha, uvechol nafshecha, uvechol meod'cha*, "with all your heart, and with all your soul, and with all your might" (Deuteronomy 6:5). God doesn't demand of us that we apportion ourselves into little pieces, some parts of which are kosher, some parts of which are acceptable, some parts of which may be public, and the rest must be hidden away. It is that hiding which is the *mum*, and a person with such a *mum* cannot serve the Holy One, and cannot stand before an imperfect community pretending to be perfect.

One can serve the Eternal only with the wholeness that comes from imperfection. With one's entire being, both positive traits and negative;

as Rashi says, *bishnei yitzarecha*, "with both your impulses." We can serve the Lord only if our entire history, our entire life, even our special needs are brought with us into the divine service. Only if our minds and our hearts and our souls are engaged passionately in the works that we do and, as we remind ourselves each *Kol Nidrei*, only if we bring with us our entire community–not just the saints but the sinners too, not just those with special needs, but those not yet with special needs.

Perhaps, then, the wholeness to which the Torah alludes is the willingness to stand in our entirety–warts and all, defects and all, special needs and all–and to offer them to God as a sacred service. Perhaps what the Torah is reminding us, then, is an insistence on a community that includes all of its members–that makes none of them invisible, that asks none of them to step outside. Perhaps only that community is a community fit to offer sacrifice that God will accept.

WE ARE CHARGED, THEN, WITH A SIMPLE BUT AWESOME TASK

Bring our entire being to the service of God and our fellow creatures. Leave no part of ourselves outside. Leave no piece of ourselves invisible. Be passionate in the service we offer. The Talmud reminds us, *Ha-Kadosh Barukh Hu liva bei*–"God wants the heart." Let us live in such a way, building communities that are welcoming and accessible, so that those we live, learn, and work with will know that they, too, are precious, and that each one of them, because of their imperfections, are truly God's children. Let us show them not to postpone encountering Torah, living mitzvot, and rejoicing in God's love until the day that they are perfect–such a day will never come. And besides, the Torah was not given to angels. We are all of us blemished; human wholeness does not come from some elusive perfection, but rather from the radical act of taking hold of our imperfections and offering even them. *Be-chol derakhekha da'ehu*–"in all your ways, know God" (Proverbs 3:6).

It is recorded in *Massekhet Sukkah* that Hillel has the audacity to speak on God's behalf. I am going to take my cue from him and muster the audacity to mistranslate Hillel. God (if not Hillel) would want it that way. "*Im ani kan, hakol kan*: 'If I am here,' says God, 'all is here.' " Who knows, but that for God to be truly present, *our* all–including the all of those with disabilities–must also be truly present.

doi: 10.1300/J095v10n03_02

ACROSS THE RELIGIOUS SPECTRUM: ORTHODOX, CONSERVATIVE AND REFORM

Jewish Theological Approaches to the Human Experience of Disability: A Primer for Rabbis and Rabbinical Students

Wallace Greene, PhD

SUMMARY. Jewish theology is firmly committed to enabling all those whom society has disenfranchised. The widow, the orphan, and the way-

Wallace Greene is Director, Jewish Educational Services, UJA Federation of Northern New Jersey. He is the Founder of Sinai Special Needs Institute, serving a special needs population from grade school through adult vocational training, and is President of the New Jersey Association of Jewish Communal Service.

[Haworth co-indexing entry note]: "Jewish Theological Approaches to the Human Experience of Disability: A Primer for Rabbis and Rabbinical Students." Greene, Wallace. Co-published simultaneously in *Journal of Religion, Disability & Health* (The Haworth Pastoral Press, an imprint of The Haworth Press, Inc.) Vol. 10, No. 3/4, 2006, pp. 9-25; and: *Jewish Perspectives on Theology and the Human Experience of Disability* (ed: Rabbi Judith Z. Abrams, and William C. Gaventa) The Haworth Pastoral Press, an imprint of The Haworth Press, Inc., 2006, pp. 9-25. Single or multiple copies of this article are available for a fee from The Haworth Document Delivery Service [1-800-HAWORTH, 9:00 a.m. - 5:00 p.m. (EST). E-mail address: docdelivery@haworthpress.com].

Available online at http://jrdh.haworthpress.com
© 2006 by The Haworth Press, Inc. All rights reserved.
doi:10.1300/J095v10n03_03

farer are but paradigms for all those who cannot fend for themselves. Rabbis and educators can be the change agents for these populations by internalizing the values that Judaism espouses. The examples chosen relate primarily to learning disabilities, but conceptually their underlying principles apply to all disabilities. doi:10.1300/J095v10n03_03 *[Article copies available for a fee from The Haworth Document Delivery Service: 1-800-HAWORTH. E-mail address: <docdelivery@haworthpress.com> Website: <http://www.HaworthPress.com> © 2006 by The Haworth Press, Inc. All rights reserved.]*

KEYWORDS. Disability, Jewish theology, theological education, learning disabilities

INTRODUCTION

There is the law, which regulates behavior, and there is theology, which seeks to understand how God relates to the world. In Judaism, they are united as one. God reveals His will via the commandments contained in the Five Books of Moses, called the Torah (literally, *instruction*). Every ritual act or moral imperative, even the narratives, reflect deeper meanings beyond the surface text. The practice of Judaism is the outward manifestation of these values. Conversely, these understandings should have an impact on the individual's *persona* as well as on her/his *praxis*.[1]

The Torah exists as two parallel forms of revelation–written and oral. The written Torah is read from a parchment scroll twice weekly and on Sabbaths and Holidays. The oral Torah is the commentary and explanations which accompanied the written document from Sinai onward. These clarifications were eventually codified and written down and became known to us as the Talmud. We understand the Torah through the teachings of the rabbis of the Talmud.[2]

God made His nature, character, and purpose, and what He would have humanity be and do, known through the revelation on Sinai which is manifest in the Torah. The Torah (both written and oral) is more than the vehicle–it is the content of revelation. There are three forms of revelation: Sinai, rabbinic interpretations, and rabbinic enactments/decrees (e.g., the Sanhedrin and its successors). This tradition will take diverse forms, since the minds of people, and consequently their ideas of God, are diverse. But so long as their minds are directed honestly to God, His inspiration will shape their ideas.[3] This would seem to be the meaning of "The words of the wise are like nails, firmly implanted, all given by one shepherd" (Ecclesiastes 12:11). Although rabbis may differ, they all draw their authority from Moses, who derived it from God.[4]

The final introductory concept concerns the immutability of the Torah. The Torah is universal as well as immutable. What is true in nature is true in religion, and what is false in science cannot be true in religion. Truth is one and indivisible. The sun, in going forth on its daily round, is fulfilling Torah as much as is a human being who worships God, as much as is a Jew when she/he performs or observes the commandments. If Torah is immutable, what about the doctrine of progress? God's Torah is immutable, be it manifested in the movements of the heavens, or in the ethics given to mankind. The standards of love, justice and truth are permanent and unchangeable. It is in the operation of those qualities among human beings, and by human beings, that development and progress are possible.

God gave man reasoning powers capable of expansion, as well as Torah. Without reason, one cannot appreciate Torah. Without Torah, one cannot utilize reason appropriately.[5] The two ideas are mutually complementary and inseparable. As reason grows, the appreciation of Torah grows–the Torah constantly reveals itself anew. The Torah is a living entity, and like all life it grows.

If there are no standards, or if the standards change, no progress is possible. Mankind cannot improve if the meaning of good and evil eventually changes. Similarly, the value of a remote, abstract idea of goodness, preserved in heaven and unattainable by humans is negligible unless we reach out to attain it, and unless we can, in the end, attain it, and that every effort brings us closer to it. A static idea of goodness, anchored in one generation is likewise limited. Torah contains the germs of expansion.[6] It is both immutable and progressive. It is ever-developing, it possesses autarky. Torah/Judaism is reality-based. It is not lifeless, conventional uniformity. The Torah expands its influence as needs arise. It develops new phases immanent in its essence.

***

Operating from the premise that the Torah's ". . . ways, are ways of pleasantness . . . " (Proverbs 3:17), and that it is " a tree of life" (Proverbs 3:18), and most significantly that "Torah scholars increase peace in the world . . . " (Talmud, *Berahot*, 64a), it is inconceivable that Judaism does not offer specific guidelines, procedures, and sensitivity to the concerns of people with disabilities. Legal aspects that relate to disability, and people with disabilities, have been studied.[7] The objective here is to present material that illustrates Judaism's understandings of disability and people with disabilities. Every legality is based on a theological position and framework. The non-legalistic portions of the Talmud have much to teach us in terms of an approach. Rabbi Joseph B. Soloveitchik, quoting his father, Rabbi Moshe Soloveitchik, taught that "The Aggadah [i.e., non-legal/narrative portions of the Talmud] is the Halakha [the binding law] of Jewish thought."[8] A search of the sources will reveal a very modern attitude towards disabilities and people with disabilities. Unfortunately, society as a whole, and to some extent the Jewish community as well, has acknowledged disability but not always put forth a cogent, systematic means to address disability (particularly within a theological framework). The power of what is socially acceptable has for too long determined the place of people with disabilities in Jewish society. Certain "infirmities" (states of embodiment) were considered socially acceptable. If one wore eyeglasses, or a hearing aid, or used a cane, there was no stigma attached to that person. If one were bald, corpulent, freckled, or pale, that, too, was acceptable. Individuals who had learning or physical disabilities, stuttered, or were otherwise labeled as "different" from societal norms were marginalized.[9] Now there is federal legislation, and many services are available, within the Jewish community.[10] Rabbis, and rabbis in training, need to know and understand the attitude of Judaism towards dealing with all forms of disabilities. They need to be able to recognize how the Torah and the Talmud viewed people with disabilities and what constitutes a disability. This understanding should lead to greater acceptance of people with disabilities, more attention to the concerns that they highlight, more integration into communal life, and more advocacy on their behalf (not just for, but *with*, them).

Synagogues, Jewish community centers, schools, and camps need to become more sensitized not just to the concerns of people with disabilities, but to what the Jewish tradition teaches about including them. This may require a bit of effort and occasional reading into the sources, but that, too, is part of the Jewish tradition. These issues are not only politically correct and in consonance with modern sensibilities, but it is the law–both federal and Jewish.

The range of disabilities referred to in classical Jewish sources is quite broad: physical, emotional, psychological, mental, and communal. Sensitivity to these conditions, awareness of them, and how Judaism views them, is the first step toward addressing them.[11]

The biblical narrative begins with God's understanding that loneliness is not good. "It is not good for man to be alone . . . " (Genesis 1:18). The making of Eve was more than just for the purpose of procreation. God's recognition of Adam's loneliness is an important lesson for contemporary times. Often individuals are alone not of their own choosing. The elderly and homebound come to mind. Those recently divorced or widowed can also be in this category. Reaching out and addressing *their* concerns may not fall under the rubric of the Disabilities Act, but in terms of being and living as Jewish, this personal and social response certainly resonates as Jewish.

The dysfunctional family life depicted in much of Genesis is also a clarion call for awareness, caring, and even intervention. There is much to learn from the text as well as from the subtext. Not all rabbis are trained clinical social workers, but they should be able to recognize the signs of trouble and be able to refer congregants for help. Jealousy, sibling rivalry, hatred, destructive behavior, malicious speech, and even malevolent actions are depicted in Genesis to teach us that even great individuals have human frailties, but more importantly, to teach us lessons about human behavior and how to avoid strife and conflict. An astute reader of these texts will be able to apply this knowledge in his/her pastoral work.

The biblical matriarchs Sarah, Rebecca, Rachel, and Hannah, mother of the prophet Samuel, as well as the mother of Samson, were all barren. Their stories and the compassion showed them by their husbands and by God are also examples of how to consider persons in these situations. While there are many viable options today for women to have a family and while, unlike the biblical narratives, not all will have their own children, we can learn how to empathize, be supportive and inclusive.

Leah, another biblical matriarch, had "weak eyes," a visual disability (Genesis 29:17), as did Isaac who was blind for part of his life (Genesis 27:1). Despite their disability, they lived productive lives. The Torah is teaching us that individuals have many contributions to make and can transcend their supposed disabilities with the proper support systems. In one community in New Jersey, a major force which drove the efforts to install an *eruv* [12] was not so much for the convenience of mothers with baby carriages, but so that a member of the congregation who became blind could walk to synagogue with his white cane. That rabbi understands the attitude of Judaism toward the people with disabilities.[13]

The patriarch Jacob had multiple disabilities which he overcame. In an overwhelmingly agricultural and farming society, Jacob was the loner, the different one who stayed inside, the one who spent his time in study and contemplation (Genesis 25:27).[14] In addition to these non-societal habits, Jacob also cooked (Genesis 25:29), and ended his life blind, and with a limp (Genesis 32:25-31; 48:8-20). He was able to respond to the challenges he faced not only with his intellect (Genesis 25:31-32; 30:42) but with the manly traits that his society valued (Genesis 29:7-10; 32:24).

One of the greatest symbols of divine advocacy on behalf of people with disabilities is Moses. His early years are quite traumatic. Moses is separated from his family as an infant, reared in an alien culture, and afflicted with a speech impediment. Yet it is he whom God chooses as the leader of the Jewish people. It is Moses whom God chooses to speak to Pharoah, not his older brother Aaron, the skilled orator (Exodus 4:14). It is Moses alone to whom God speaks directly (Deuteronomy 34:10). This notion of leadership focuses on strength of character, not physical characteristics. It teaches us that people with disabilities are to be included in communal roles.

People who have disabilities may be hesitant to assume such public leadership roles, but no more so than others. Moses declared his reluctance on several occasions (Exodus 2:11; 13; 4:1; 10; 13). There are other cases in the Bible of leadership roles taken by individuals with a variety of disabilities.[15] Judaism teaches against discrimination.

It seems clear that Judaism, from its earliest inception, enunciated the view that the person with a disability was not to be exploited, demeaned, or otherwise discriminated against.[16] Judaism teaches that a disability is not to be equated with a lack of intelligence or understanding. Therefore it is forbidden to curse the deaf (Leviticus 19:14). Obviously a deaf person cannot hear such a curse, however, we are being taught a lesson in sensitivity. The Torah legislates such behavior to teach that deafness does not imply lack of comprehension. A similar idea is put forth in the law prohibiting one from placing a stumbling block before the blind (ibid.). Here, too, the Torah goes beyond the obvious and makes what to us may seem common sense into a legal requirement. Apparently, human behavior in the ancient world was not always so predisposed.[17] The need for this legislation is underscored by ". . . and you shall fear your God, I am the Lord" (ibid.), since left to their own human reasoning, mankind may not come to this conclusion on their own. The message is clear–we are responsible for the welfare of all members of our community and may not do anything to undermine them.[18]

The Torah stipulates that it is the heritage of *all* Jews (Deuteronomy 33:4). Judaism is inclusive and no Jew is to be excluded. An inheritance belongs to heirs to use and dispose of as they wish. A heritage, on the other hand, belongs to the generations and must be preserved intact. That is our mandate[19] since all generations were said to be present at Sinai (Deuteronomy 29:13-14).

There are a number of philosophical/theological foundations for a Jewish value system which mandates that we include people with disabilities. We need to move beyond seeing people with disabilities as needy, and toward a view that all people have needs. This model stresses interdependency as a central characteristic of life and society.

Reference was already made to the biblical injunction against placing a stumbling block before the blind (Leviticus 19:14). Beyond the obvious, literal intent of the verse is a dispute among the sages. Some felt that there was no need to have a special law against causing blind people to stumble since there are a sufficient number of laws protecting all individuals from malicious harm.[20] Others believe that biblical verses maintain their literal meaning even when the oral tradition expands and adds additional meanings. Suffice it to say that "blind" is understood to mean any person or group that is in any way vulnerable. It is prohibited to do them any harm. Conversely, one must be proactive to prevent harm from coming to them. Nechama Leibowitz, the famous Israeli Bible teacher (20th century), suggests a very broad understanding of this verse:

> . . . the Torah teaches us that even by sitting at home doing nothing, by complete passivity and divorcement from society, one cannot shake off responsibility for what is transpiring in the world at large, for the iniquity, violence, and evil there. By not protesting, [and taking action] . . . you have become responsible for any harm arising therefrom, and have violated the prohibition "Thou shalt not place a stumbling block before the blind . . . "[21]

With this understanding, it is not difficult to suggest that the following services (among others) fall under this rubric:

- Make all buildings handicapped-accessible inside and out.
- Make available large print books, prayer books, Jewish texts, and Bibles.
- Provide Jewish books in Braille and recordings for adults and children.[22]
- Create and support special schools and programs for people with disabilities.[23]

- Develop and support Jewish/kosher adult residential programs for people who have developmental disabilities.[24]
- Guarantee (kosher) Meals on Wheels for those who need it.
- Provide sign language instruction/programs for the Jewish deaf.

The seemingly simple verse prohibiting the placement of stumbling blocks before the blind is actually a succinct statement encompassing many important concepts. It is an admonition not to be passive, a clarion call to action demanding that the Jewish community do everything possible to welcome and include all people. It is a fundamental principle on a par with "Love your fellow human being as yourself" (Leviticus 19:18).

Another theological underpinning which militates for action and advocacy for people with disabilities is the Jewish concept of *imitatio Dei*. Just as God is kind and merciful, so, too, should we imitate His ways. He is concerned for all people. Why would this not refer to people with disabilities?[25] The Jewish communal leadership needs to open their eyes and hearts and make these concerns more of a priority. Rabbis can play an important role in this process. Like the prophets of old, rabbis can exhort their communities to remove that which covers their hearts to be open to these initiatives. Those who are stubborn and refuse to see the theological imperatives inherent in advocating for people with disabilities might qualify as having an uncircumcised heart.[26]

There is another biblical imperative pregnant with meaning which is germane to our inquiry. ". . . neither shall you stand idly by the blood of your neighbor, I am the Lord" (Leviticus 19:16). This is understood by the rabbis of the Talmud and codified by Maimonides to mean that anyone who is in physical proximity, or even knows about someone in peril, is duty bound to save that person. If someone is able and does not act to save this person, he/she has transgressed the commandment of ". . . neither shall you stand idly by the blood of your neighbor." Saving someone in danger can be done in person or by hiring others. Every life is considered sacrosanct as is the quality of life. Loss of even one life is considered as destroying the entire world. Conversely, saving one person is like preserving the entire world.[27] Here, too, we are expanding the Good Samaritan law to include individuals with disabilities. This is not mere homiletics but is integral to the conceptual understanding of this commandment.

Although many individuals with disabilities live full and productive lives, those without a support system experience isolation from relationships. The Bible recognizes that certain disabilities render a person helpless in many ways and subject to exploitation.[28] That is why the Bible warns against exploiting them.[29] Limitations based on physical disabilities are symbolically interpreted as being the equivalent of death. "He has made me to dwell in darkness as those who have long been dead" (Lamentations 3:6).[30] Hence, the connection to the legal imperative of saving those whose lives are imperiled is valid. A bystander is required to go to great personal effort, even to incur financial loss and hardship, to save someone's life. Since blindness is a natural metaphor for oppression and injustice, [31] rabbis have the opportunity to clarify the vision of their communities regarding people with disabilities.

The verse of not standing idly by while someone is in danger is understood by the Rabbis of the Talmud to obligate the bystander to go to extraordinary lengths to save the victim–even to the extent of hiring help. Along comes a second verse ". . . and you shall restore it to him" (Deuteronomy 22:2) which broadens this imperative. Whereas the duty to rescue (derived from the law of returning lost articles) would have been limited to one's personal ability, the latter verse encompasses the duty to come to the assistance of one who is in distress but not necessarily in peril.[32] Even if peril is not at hand, the obligation to enter into a rescue operation is not diminished.

According to Maimonides, one who violates these prohibitions is not flogged because his/her breach involves no overt action (aye there's the rub). However, the offense is quite serious nevertheless.[33] Given the foregoing analysis, there is no reason why the Jewish community and its leadership should not be held accountable for not coming to the rescue of those who are indeed in peril and who are in need of our help.

Narrative passages in the Talmud may not always be taken literally, but they must always be taken seriously. A survey of all the relevant materials related to the various forms of disabilities would be beyond a volume monograph. A number of rabbinic sources related to dealing with the special needs student will suffice to make the case that Jewish theology supports the full inclusion of people with disabilities. It should also advocate for and with them in society.

The primary source which describes the origin of universal public Jewish education, credits Rabbi Joshua ben Gamla (d. 69/70 C.E.) with this innovation. Aside from establishing a school system, he developed pedagogic methodologies far advanced for his time. He limited class size for one teacher, required team teaching in larger classes, mandated paraprofessionals when necessary, and made each town responsible for funding the schools and paying salaries.[34] His enactments were later codified into the canons of Jewish law.[35] The obligation to educate children Jewishly was thus transferred from the home to the school. Since not every parent was a competent teacher, nor had the time, ability, knowledge, and patience to instruct, this was a significant departure from tradition. The Torah requires parents to teach their children (Deuteronomy 6:7). R. Joshua ben Gamla placed this obligation squarely on the community, *in loco parentis*.[36]

Parents were (and still are) often unable to provide a Jewish education for their children. While this is unfortunately true for the general school population, it is even more serious for the child with special needs. In these cases, parents who want to provide a Jewish education for their special needs child often are unable to find a suitable and appropriate program. Programs exist in the public school system for their special needs students. It is the law. As will be demonstrated, it is also the law in Judaism. But this law is usually observed more in its breach than in its observance. The Jewish community lacks the central authority to make anything compulsory. There are a number of programs throughout the U.S. for synagogue schools and day schools. It is by no means universal. When one considers that 10%-15% of any school population has some form of a developmental disability, these programs should be in every school in every community.

Some parents move to another state to find an appropriate program for their Jewish special needs child. Many opt to stay put and rationalize that the special needs child probably couldn't handle a second curriculum, or are content with some form of minimal tutelage. When this happens, these children get all sorts of negative messages, especially when there are siblings who are receiving a Jewish education. This should not be allowed to happen to any Jewish child today. Among the reasons given for the destruction of Jerusalem in 586 B.C.E. was ". . . because children did not attend school, and loitered in the streets."[37]

When Rabbi Joshua ben Gamla issued his edict, he included all children. He didn't set up a system for "special" children but meant for them to be educated along with the other students. Today this is called mainstreaming. The Talmud quotes the scholar Rav who taught that if a student is having difficulty, place that student next to one who is doing well. This, too, is codified as Jewish law.[38] The original thinking of the Sages was to encourage heterogeneous classes. Obviously, at some point the more talented students would be separated to pursue higher studies. However, the major thrust of this inclusion argument is that every child is capable of some learning. Every child can master something and ought not to be singled out or discriminated against.[39] As early as the Bible itself we are admonished to "Train the child according to his ability. . . " (Proverbs 22:6). The Sages understood that for every thousand students who begin the study of the Bible, maybe one hundred will advance to the study of Mishna. Of that group, maybe ten will master the Talmud, and from them one may emerge as a great scholar.[40] Not only is the entire enterprise worthwhile in order to produce that one out of a thousand, but in the process, the other nine hundred and ninety-nine are productively studying on their level.

What emerges from this position is that every Jew has his/her own share in the Torah. It is irrelevant if that portion is the biblical text, the Mishna or the Talmud. No one may legitimately deprive anyone else of their share in Torah. The Jewish liturgy reflects this notion in the oft repeated phrase ". . . grant us our portion in Your Torah. . . ." Every Jew has an obligation to study *his/her* portion based on time, inclination, and ability. Everyone's portion is equally valid. Even if one person is on a higher level, that person is where he/she belongs. In reality, stealing a bicycle is no less of a crime than stealing a car. Theft is theft. The same applies to one's share/portion of Torah. It is morally repugnant and a flagrant violation of Torah values to deprive any child of his/her share of Torah because some might consider it less valid or compelling.

The Torah teaches that "Moses charged us with the Torah as the heritage for the congregation of Jacob [i.e., all Jews]" (Deuteronomy 33:4). No class of Jews is singled out for omission. Therefore, the Talmud comments that one who deprives someone from studying Torah is guilty of stealing.[41] Throughout Jewish history there have always been study groups available on every level. Groups gather to study the weekly Torah portion, there is a *hevra tehillim* for the recitation and study of Psalms, a *hevra mishnayot* for the study of Mishna, *hevra shas* for the study of Talmud, etc. Since Torah study is a cardinal principle of Judaism, opportunities exist on all levels so that no child or adult is excluded or disenfranchised. Just as the Jewish community must provide schools in general, it has an identical obligation to guarantee that children with learning differences have a Jewish education as well.[42] This is the meaning of Isaiah 54:13: "And *all* your children shall be students of the Lord, and great shall be the happiness of your children."

The Jewish theology of inclusion also reflects an understanding of how students who have developmental disabilities feel. The Talmud records that Rabbi Pereidah (3rd century) had a student who required that lessons be repeated four hundred (i.e., very many) times before he grasped it. It is interesting to note that (a) Rabbi Pereidah, a great scholar, did not feel that teaching such a student was beneath him, and (b) he actually took the time to work with this student until he mastered his lessons. He did not give up on him even though it required much effort. Once it happened that Rabbi Pereidah had an important appointment immediately after his session with this student. He taught the student his lesson four hundred times, and yet he still did not comprehend the material. When he asked what was bothering him, the student replied that since he knew that Rabbi Pereidah had to leave right after the session, he focused (obsessed) on that, not knowing when his teacher would be leaving, and therefore his attention was not fully focused on the lesson. He kept on thinking, will my teacher leave now, will he leave now, etc. Rabbi Pereidah responded that he shouldn't worry, that he wouldn't leave until the student mastered his daily lesson, and he remained to teach him another four hundred times. Such devotion, kindness, and empathy did not go unrewarded. A Heavenly Voice proclaimed that Rabbi Pereidah could claim an extra four hundred (i.e., many) years of life or that he and his generation would be guaranteed a place in the World to Come. He chose the World to Come and was granted both.[43] This narrative is included in the Talmudic text as an example and model of the qualities of a good teacher. It is not unlike the educational culture of Japan which insists that there are no poor students, only poor teachers.

When the Talmud exhorts teachers to make sure that their students understand their lessons (*Sanhedrin* 91b) one might think that this refers to a class of "regular" students. Not so, writes Rabbi Shmuel Edels (17th century), known as the MaHaRShA, in his commentary *ad loc*:

> [This means that a teacher who doesn't make sure his students understand the lesson] . . . is not teaching the way that Rabbi Pereidah did. . . . and by preventing a student from learning [by not reviewing as often as necessary] until the student is fluent the teacher is thereby stealing that student's heritage [i.e., Torah]. A teacher might say that a certain student is not up to it and incapable of learning. If so, that teacher is robbing the student of his ancestral heritage.

Not only is it incumbent upon us to teach *all* youngsters, even those with less ability, but we must endeavor to find modalities where they can learn and succeed. This is exemplified in the Talmud by Rabbi Haninah. There is a legal concept that the verses of the Torah must be recited as they were written, i.e., in a complete sentence. Rabbi Haninah was frustrated by this ruling since the children he was teaching could not learn an entire verse, and sought permission to break up the verses to make them easier to remember.[44] He could have given up, but he persevered on behalf of his students and eventually found a way that was acceptable. Breaking down the learning into component parts did not achieve prominence until Benjamin Bloom's taxonomy was published in 1956. Rabbi Haninah intuitively understood this in the second century!

Throughout history, Jewish scholars have made not only education, but education of all children a priority. In the eighteenth century, Rabbi Joseph Teomim (known as the Pri Megadim for his monumental commentary on the Shulhan Arukh) published a unique Bible. In Hebrew, all verbs have a three letter root form which appears in all tenses. In order to make the text more understandable, the regular text appears in outline form while the root letters of all verbs are solid, e.g., take the English word **EAT**ery, meaning restaurant. The root letters E A T are solid while the E R Y are outlined. Recognition of the root letters makes comprehension easier and aids as well as a contextual clue.[45]

Teachers need to be creative in order to find the right vehicles for their students' success. If a teacher says that he/she is not a publisher, then he/she is not really a teacher either. Sometimes it is difficult to focus on the concerns of every single student, even in the best of situations. When this occurs, there is also a precedent to establish special classes for those who require more individualized attention. The community of Altona even passed a communal ordinance to this effect in 1808.[46]

The goal of all education, not just that of special needs students, is to find the best way(s) for them to access knowledge in the least frustrating manner. It all comes back to wise King Solomon in Proverbs 22:6 who instructed us to teach each child according to his/her ability. This concept is elaborated upon by Rabbi Shmuel Edels (17th century):

> Teach the student gently, as if you were handfeeding an ox and not
> . . . the way that [some animals]are force-fed.[47]

Once we have recognized our obligation to provide proper and adequate instruction to all children, we must then provide appropriately trained faculty. There are many universities offering degrees in special education, but there is a dearth of graduate level programs dealing specifically with the special needs child in a Jewish school environment. Not only is it important for these teachers to have mastered content and approach, but somehow we need to make sure that these special teachers have the right disposition. These teachers need to be exceptionally organized, friendly, and patient.[48] As one illustration, we can read in *Sefer Hasidim* (ca. 1200, Germany) as follows:

> There was once a student who stuttered and it took him quite a while before he managed to get a word out of his mouth, and when the others laughed at him he became [even more] frustrated. His teacher told him not to ask questions [orally] in class but to write them down or wait until after class and he would explain any difficulties he was having.[49]

Perhaps the definitive characterization of the Jewish theological position vis-à-vis learning disabilities is contained in the following narrative:

> Rabbi Yohanan said: Each of the forty days that Moses was on Mt. Sinai, God taught him the entire Torah, but each day he forgot it. Finally, God gave it to him as a gift. Why did this [process] take [until] forty days? In order to encourage slow learners.[50]

When teachers are able to make their instruction a "gift" to their students it is valued that much more. Moses had the best teacher. Yet even He had to modify the way He taught. Moses became, in turn, the teacher of the Jewish people.

Jews have received a mandate to be concerned with every individual in society. This concern is not to be articulated by way of maudlin condescension but, rather, by way of justice. In Judaism, the relationship between justice and love is a central and crucial idea. To the Jew, "justice" is that condition which makes possible the appropriate interaction between people, irrespective of their emotional stance towards one another. The just thing must be done. . . . It may be nice to love everyone, says Judaism, but failure to do so must not be reflected in action. Hence "Justice, justice shall you pursue" (Deuteronomy 16:20) not "love, love shall you feel." Why? Since justice can be articulated in action, just actions can be mandated. Love is an emotion, and emotions cannot be legislated. Hence, Judaism demands *just* treatment of all members of society irrespective of how one may *feel* about them. This, then, is the . . . normative Jewish attitude toward the treatment of any individual, handicapped or otherwise: a mature attitude of meaningful concern unencumbered and unmarred by emotions, either of condescension or pity or even favoritism. It bespeaks a need to deal with concerns; dislike or aversion is no excuse for inaction.[51]

NOTES

1. See *Sefer HaHinukh* (Spain, 13th century) Chavel edition (Jerusalem, 1966) #285, p. 366. Actions affect thought which shapes future behavior. The symbolism of the commandments and what they represent are intended to make a lasting impression upon those who observe these rituals with the appropriate understanding of their underlying principles.

2. See *The Epistle of R. Sherira Gaon* (11th cent.), trans. R. Nosson Dovid Rabinovich (Jerusalem, 1988) for a history of the Oral Law. See also R. Zvi Hirsch Chajes (19th cent.), *The Student's Guide Through the Mishna*, trans. Jacob Schachter (New York, 1960).

3. See Abraham Joshua Heschel (20th cent.), *God in Search of Man* (NY, 1955), p. 198. According to Heschel, revelation represents an event in which God communicates His teachings and concern for man. See also Rabbi Joseph B. Soloveitchik (20th cent.) "Lonely Man of Faith" *TRADITION* (VII:2, 1965), p. 46. "Man in dialogue with God re-experiences the rendezvous with God in which the covenant originated." In other words, study is a form of contemporary revelation. See also R. Chayyim Volozin (19th cent.), *Nefesh HaChayyim* (Vilna, 1824) *passim* for similar sentiments.

4. See *Pesiqta Rabbati* (6-7th cent.), 8a-8b.

5. See *Avot* 3:21.

6. See *Midrash Tanhuma, (4th Cent.),Yitro 11, 124a-b.*

7. See Tzvi C. Marx, *Disability in Jewish Law* (2002); and Hefziba Lifshitz and Joav Merrick, "Jewish Law and the Definition of Mental Retardation: The Status of People with Intellectual Disability Within Jewish Law," *Journal of Religion, Disability & Health* 5:1 (2001), pp. 39-52.

8. Rabbi Joseph B. Soloveitchik, from a transcription of his annual *yahrzeit shiur* [Yiddish] delivered on 4 Sh'vat, 5730 (1970) at Yeshiva University in New York.

9. One could add to this list those who were single, divorced, or lefthanded.

10. An internet search will yield many resources in many communities which deal with an array of disabilities. Unfortunately, there are more people with disabilities than there are programs. It is far from being the norm and these services should exist in every community.

11. See Morton K. Siegel, "Seminal Jewish Attitudes Toward the Handicapped," *Journal of Religion, Disability & Health* 5:1 (2001), pp. 29-38.

12. An *eruv* is a rabbinic device which demarcates the boundaries of a Jewish community via telephone wires or other markers. By thus symbolically enclosing the area it becomes one domain and Orthodox Jews are thereby allowed to carry, wheel baby carriages, etc. within its precincts. Most large, and many smaller Jewish communities today have a *eruv*. See *New York Times*, October 25, 2002, "Symbolic Enclosure Is Allowed, Judges Rule," Section B, Page 5, Column 4.

13. Cf. Rivka Glaubman and Hefziba Lifshitz, "Ultra-orthodox Jewish Teachers' Self-efficacy and Willingness for Inclusion of Pupils with Special Needs," *European Journal of Special Needs Education* (2001, 16:3) pp. 207-223; and H. Lifshitz and M.L. Naor, "Student Teachers' Willingness to Mainstream Pupils with Special Needs in Relation to Track and Severity of Disability," *International Journal of Rehabilitation Research* (24:2001), pp. 143-148.

14. See commentary of RaShI *ad loc.*

15. See for example Ehud ben Gera (Judges 3:15) who was lefthanded; and Jepthah (Judges 11:1-11) who was illegitimate.

16. Legal limitations, however, do exist. A deaf person, due to his objective limitations cannot perform certain legal functions. A person with diminished capacity is exempt from certain responsibilities. These exclusions are based on competency, not castigation.

17. See *Classical Studies 150W Archive* 1998, *Greek and Roman Private Life* in the *Department of Classical Studies*, College of William and Mary, posted by Professor, *W.E. Hutton*. When physically or mentally impaired children were born, the parents were faced with a difficult decision. They could raise their children who had disabilities to try and reach adulthood, or they could dispose of the infant by either killing the child or leaving it exposed to the elements to die. This act of killing newborn children is known as infanticide and was a common practice in the ancient world, especially in Athens and Sparta (Edwards, 1). There are only a few ancient sources that discuss the topic of infanticide; these coming from Plato, Aristotle, Plutarch, and Soranus. Plato describes a utopia of sorts in his *Republic* and states that the offspring of healthy parents were raised, while the progeny from inferior parents were secreted away (460C). Aristotle takes a more drastic and harsh view stating, "As to exposing or rearing the children born, let there be a law that no deformed child shall be reared" (*Politics,* 1335B). In his account of Lycurgus, Plutarch makes reference to the Spartan system of examining and rearing newborn children. The newborns were examined by the elders of society and if the babies were deemed to be healthy and strong, they were ordered to be reared. If the child was deformed or weak, they were sent to a ravine at the foot of a mountain to die. Spartans believed that one with a disability from birth would be disadvantageous to the state. The final example from ancient sources comes from Soranus' *Gynecology*. A set of criteria was listed to decide whether a child was worth rearing (2.6). Some of these requirements were the mother's health during the pregnancy, length of pregnancy, the strength of the child's cry, and having complete body parts.

18. Morton Siegel, "Seminal Jewish Attitudes Toward the Handicapped," *Journal of Religion, Disability & Health* 5:1 (2001), pp. 29-38, compares the treatment of lepers in the ancient world to the humane treatment in Judaism of one afflicted by *tzara'at*. Rabbi Samson Rafael Hirsch (19th cent.), in his Commentary to The Torah on Leviticus Chapter 13, shows definitively that the symptoms of *tzara'at* are far different from those of leprosy. Cf. the Stone edition of *The Chumash* (ArtScroll), pp. 609-10.

19. The legal obligation to take care of those in need extends even to the dead. In fact, it is the highest form of a kindness since it can never be repaid. See *Jerusalem Talmud, Pe'ah* 1:1; and *Midrash Tanhuma* (Buber), *V'yehi,* 107a.

20. See Rabbi Joseph Babad (19th cent.) *Minhat Hinukh,* 232:4.

21. See Nechama Leibowitz, *Studies in Leviticus* (Jerusalem,1983).

22. Available from Jewish Heritage for the Blind, The Jewish Braille Institute of America, and The Library of Congress. The Jewish Braille Institute of America was founded in 1931 by The National Federation of (Reform) Temple Sisterhoods.

23. Fortunately, many such programs exist, but unfortunately not in every community.

24. Such Jewish adult residential programs exist in a number of communities for adults with special needs. There is even a residential therapeutic program for those with addictions and compulsive disorders. These residences should be in every community.

25. See *Mechilta* to Exodus 15:2; *Talmud Shabbat* 133b; *Sotah* 14a and parallels; and Maimonides, *Sefer HaMizvot,* Positive Commandment #8.

26. See Jeremiah 9:26, and Ezekiel 44:7;9. Cf. NT Acts 7:51.

27. See R. Moses Maimonides (12th cent.), *Mishneh Torah, Torts: Murder and Preservation of Life* 1:14;16. The analogy to destroying/preserving the entire world is based on the idea that at one time Adam represented all of humanity. Cf. Talmud, *Avot of Rabbi Nathan*, Version I:31:45b-46a.

28. See Samuel II:5:6; Isaiah 35:5-6; Jeremiah 31:8; and Deuteronomy 28:29.

29. See Leviticus 19:14; Deuteronomy 28:18; and Job 29:15.

30. See Talmud, *Nedarim* 64b.

31. See Deuteronomy 28:28-29; Isaiah 59:9-10, and Lamentations 4:14.

32. See Talmud, *Sanhedrin* 73a.

33. See n. 27 above.

34. See Talmud, *Babba Batra* 21a.

35. Maimonides, *Laws of Teaching Torah* 2:1, and R. Jacob ben Asher, *Tur Shulhan Arukh, Yoreh Deah* 145:7.

36. See comments of Rabbi Meir Simha HaCohen, *Or Sameah* on Maimonides, *Laws of Teaching Torah* 1:2.

37. Talmud, *Shabbat* 119b.

38. Talmud, *Babba Batra* 21a, and *Shulhan Arukh, Yoreh Deah* 245:9.

39. See Renee Nussbaum (unpublished Ph.D. dissertation), *Broken Promises Fulfilled: A Partial-Inclusion Program for Students with Severe Learning Disabilities at The Middle School Level*, Walden University (November, 2002).

40. See *Midrash Leviticus Rabbah* 2:1 and *Midrash Ecclesiastes Rabbah* 7:49.

41. Talmud, *Sanhedrin* 91b.

42. Rabbi Moses Feinstein (20th cent.), *Responsa Igrot Moshe, Yoreh Deah* IV:29.

43. Talmud, *Eruvin* 54b. Cf. Talmud *Megillah* 27b. Students asked Rabbi Pereidah to what he attributed his long life. He answered that he was always the first to attend the study hall. Either he was extremely modest about God's promise to him, or was not aware of what had been granted to him. See *Tosafot ad loc.*

44. Talmud, *Ta'anit* 27b. See comment of RaShI *ad loc.* Rabbi Haninah kept on going back to his teacher and was persistent until he was granted permission to break up the verses. The phrase RaShI uses is "until he gave *me* permission" indicating that Rabbi Haninah felt that this was *his* problem, i.e., his students' problem became his problem, showing the level of his empathy.

45. This text is in the possession of Dr. Aharon Fried, one of the pioneers in the field of Jewish Learning Disabilities.

46. See Simcha Assaf, *Sources for the History of Jewish Education* (Heb.) (Jerusalem, 1943), "Communal Ordinances of Altona-Hamburg" 2:14.

47. Commentary to Talmud, *Babba Batra* 21a.

48. See Talmud, *Ta'anit* 7b-8a; Maimonides, *Laws of Teaching Torah* 4:4-5.

49. See *Sefer Hasidim*, ed. by J. Wistinetzki (Frankfort a.M., 1924) #785, p. 197.

50. See Jerusalem Talmud, *Horayot*, end.

51. See Morton K. Siegel, "Seminal Jewish Attitudes Toward the Handicapped," *Journal of Religion, Disability & Health* 5:1 (2001), p. 33.

doi: 10.1300/J095v10n03_03

The Participation of Jews Who Are Blind in the Torah Service

Rabbi Daniel S. Nevins, MA

SUMMARY. Jews who are blind are generally obligated to observe the commandments, even those which apparently require vision. They may certainly lead prayer services and chant from the Haftarah for the congregation. Torah reading is a special case since it must be performed directly from a kosher scroll. while adaptive devices may eventually allow a blind person to read directly from the parchment, at this point there are three options for Jews who are blind to read Torah: (1) To receive an aliyah and repeat the words after the sighted reader; (2) to serve as meturgamon, the simultaneous translator of the text (like the Talmudic Rav Yosef, who was blind); (2) chant the maftir section from a braille Bible after it is chanted by a sighted reader as shevii. This responsum

---

Rabbi Daniel S. Nevins serves on the Committee on Jewish Law & Standards. He is Rabbi of Adat Shalom Synagogue in Farmington Hills Michigan, where he has served since his ordination at The Jewish Theological Seminary of America in 1994. Rabbi Nevins received his undergraduate degree in history from Harvard College in 1989. He currently serves on The Rabbinical Assembly's Executive Council. His personal web page is: www.rabbinevins.org

This paper was approved by the CJLS on January 15, 2003, by a vote of sixteen in favor (16-0-0). Voting in favor: Rabbis Kassel Abelson, Ben Zion Bergman, Elliot N. Dorff, Paul Drazen, Robert Fine, Baruch Frydman-Kohl, Myron S. Geller, Vernon H. Kurtz, Daniel Nevins, Hillel Norry, Paul Plotkin, Joseph Prouser, Mayer Rabinowitz, Joel E. Rembaum, Joel Roth, and Elie Kaplan Spitz.

[Haworth co-indexing entry note]: "The Participation of Jews Who Are Blind in the Torah Service." Nevins, Rabbi Daniel S. Co-published simultaneously in *Journal of Religion, Disability & Health* (The Haworth Pastoral Press, an imprint of The Haworth Press, Inc.) Vol. 10, No. 3/4, 2006, pp. 27-52; and: *Jewish Perspectives on Theology and the Human Experience of Disability* (ed: Rabbi Judith Z. Abrams, and William C. Gaventa) The Haworth Pastoral Press, an imprint of The Haworth Press, Inc., 2006, pp. 27-52. Single or multiple copies of this article are available for a fee from The Haworth Document Delivery Service [1-800-HAWORTH, 9:00 a.m. - 5:00 p.m. (EST). E-mail address: docdelivery@haworthpress.com].

Available online at http://jrdh.haworthpress.com
doi:10.1300/J095v10n03_04

was approved by the CJLS on January 15, 2003 by a vote of 16 in favor (16-0-0). The responsum includes technical information [Jewish Law] regarding the inclusion of Jews who are blind in the Torah service. doi:10.1300/J095v10n03_04 *[Article copies available for a fee from The Haworth Document Delivery Service: 1-800-HAWORTH. E-mail address: <docdelivery@ haworthpress.com> Website: <http://www.HaworthPress.com> © 2006 by The Haworth Press, Inc. All rights reserved.]*

KEYWORDS. Blind, suma, iveir, Torah reader, aliyah, dignity

שאלה:[1]

Can a person who is blind read Torah by memorizing the *parshah*, or by placing a scanner on top of the Torah text that would translate the text into braille?

תשובה:[2]

לֹא־תְקַלֵּל חֵרֵשׁ וְלִפְנֵי עִוֵּר לֹא תִתֵּן מִכְשֹׁל וְיָרֵאתָ מֵּאֱלֹקֶיךָ אֲנִי ה': ויקרא יט, יד.

Do not curse the deaf nor shall you place a stumbling block before the blind; you shall revere your God–I am Adonai.

(Leviticus 19:14)

Throughout Jewish history, Jews who are blind have functioned as full members of the Jewish community, and in many cases, as spiritual and educational leaders too. In contrast to many ancient societies which scorned and persecuted people with disabilities, Judaism has taught us to see the infinite worth of human life and to preserve the safety and dignity of all people. One measure of a person's dignity is the extent to which he or she is included in the ritual expectations of his or her community.

There is a substantial halakhic literature regarding the obligations of Jews who are blind to observe the mitzvot and their ability to fulfill various ritual requirements on behalf of themselves, their families and the congregation.[3] In this responsum, we will review the debate about the general obligation of Jews who are blind to observe the commandments, and then the specific literature addressing their receiving an *aliyah* to the Torah, as well as reading Torah for the congregation. This paper will not address all aspects of ritual practice, but will touch on specific mitzvot which have been the basis for Jewish case law on the blind. Dr. Avraham Steinberg lists twenty-eight mitzvot (e.g., ברכת המלך, the blessing upon seeing a king) that would seem to require vision for which the blind are nevertheless obligated, as well as fifteen mitzvot for which their physical disability prevents participation. Our question is into which category the various roles of the Torah service fall.

ARE BLIND JEWS OBLIGATED TO KEEP THE MITZVOT?

The foundation text for our question is a *sugya* found in *Bava Kamma* 86b-87a. The anonymous Mishnah (8:1) states that:

הַמְבַיֵּשׁ אֶת הֶעָרוֹם, הַמְבַיֵּשׁ אֶת הַסּוּמָא, וְהַמְבַיֵּשׁ אֶת הַיָּשֵׁן, חַיָּב.

He who humiliates one who is naked, blind or asleep is liable.

In this text, three classes of victims are qualified for indemnification. Yet what if these individuals were not the victims, but rather the perpetrators? The Mishnah states that one who is *asleep* is not liable for humiliation that he caused, וְיָשֵׁן שֶׁבִּיֵּשׁ, פָּטוּר. It does not, however, indicate whether a *blind* (or a naked) person is liable for causing humiliation to others. The lack of a parallel exemption in the Mishnah for Jews who are blind is understood to imply[4] that they are indeed liable for any humiliation which they might cause to others.[5]

In the Gemara, Rabbi Yehudah is cited disagreeing with the *Stam Mishnah*,[6] stating that, סומא אין לו בושת, literally, "a blind man has no disgrace." At first blush, this remark seems to mean that Rabbi Yehudah exempts sighted people for the humiliation of the blind! However, Rashi and Tosafot understand Rabbi Yehudah's statement to disagree only with the Mishnah's implication that people who are blind are themselves liable should they humiliate others. As Tosafot notes,

דמודה רבי יהודה דמבייש את הסומא חייב,

"for Rabbi Yehudah agrees [with the Mishnah] that one who humiliates the blind is liable."[7]

The true question is why Rabbi Yehudah exempts Jews who are blind for damage done to others, and why the Mishnah holds them liable. The Talmud records,

וכן היה רבי יהודה פוטרו מכל מצות האמורות בתורה,

"and so too did Rabbi Yehudah exempt [the blind] from all mitzvot mentioned in the Torah." Through the use of *gezeirah shava* and other interpretive techniques, the Gemara shows how Rabbi Yehudah's exemption of Jews who are blind from various liabilities reflected his broader exemption of the blind from *all* mitzvot.

From this *sugya* in *Bava Kamma*, we learn that Jews who are blind are generally bound to the mitzvot according to the Mishnah. Although the Halakha was established in accordance with the teaching of the Mishnah, substantial confusion on the topic apparently reigned in the subsequent generations, as indicated by the statement of Rav Yosef, who was blind:[8]

אמר רב יוסף: מריש הוה אמינא, מאן דאמר הלכה כר' יהודה, דאמר: סומא פטור מן
המצות, קא עבידנא יומא טבא לרבנן. מ"ט? דהא לא מפקדינא וקא עבידנא מצוות.
והשתא דשמעיתא להא דר' חנינא דאמר ר' חנינא: גדול מצווה ועושה ממי שאינו מצווה
ועושה, מאן דאמר לי דאין הלכה כרבי יהודה, עבידנא יומא טבא לרבנן. מ"ט? דכי
מפקדינא אית לי אגרא טפי.

Rav Yosef said, I initially said that if someone would teach the law like Rabbi Yehudah, who stated "the blind are exempt from the mitzvot," I would make a feast for the rabbis [in his honor]. Why? For I am not commanded, but nevertheless I perform the mitzvot. But now that I have heard that said by Rabbi Hanina, "Greater is he who is commanded and performs [mitzvot] than is one who is not commanded but still performs [the mitzvot]," whoever can teach that the law is *not* like Rabbi Yehudah, I will make a feast for the rabbis [in his honor]. Why? If I am commanded, then I shall have a greater reward!

We do not learn the fate of Rav Yosef's dinner party. Indeed, we are left to question whether the סומא has a general requirement, or a general exemption, for observing the commandments. Thus it is significant to learn on *Pesachim* 116b that Rav Yosef and his blind colleague Rav Sheshet each observed Passover and apparently recited the relevant blessings on behalf of their sighted guests:

אמר רב אחא בר יעקב: סומא פטור מלומר הגדה. כתיב הכא בעבור זה וכתיב התם בנו
זה. מה להלן- פרט לסומא, אף כאן - פרט לסומין. איני? והאמר מרימר: שאלתינהו לרבנן
דבי רב יוסף: מאן דאמר אגדתא בי רב יוסף? אמרו: רב יוסף. מאן דאמר אגדתא בי רב
ששת? אמרו: רב ששת.

Rav Acha bar Yaakov said, the blind are exempt from reciting the Haggadah. It is written here [in the Seder, citing Exodus 13:8] "because of *this*,"[9] and it is written there [Deut. 21:20, regarding the rebellious son] "*this*, our son."[10] Just as there–to exclude the blind, so too here, to exclude the blind. Really? Did not Mareimar relate, we asked the rabbis from the school of Rav Yosef, "who recited the Haggadah in the house of Rav Yosef?" They said, "Rav Yosef." Who recited the Haggadah in the house of Rav Sheshet?" They said, "Rav Sheshet."

Rav Acha bar Yaakov's *gezeira shava* notwithstanding, these rabbis acted as obligated Jews in reciting the Haggadah and were apparently also the agents of their guests.[11] At the very least, the story indicates that Jews who are blind may accept upon themselves the obligation to observe the commandments.[12]

Another sugya on *Beitzah* 16b relates that a student who was blind was held liable to prepare an ערוב תבשילין[13] by his teacher Mar Shmuel:

ההוא סמיא דהוה מסדר מתניתא קמיה דמר שמואל, חזייה דהוה עציב: אמר ליה: אמאי עציבת? - אמר ליה: דלא אותיבי ערובי תבשילין. - אמר ליה: סמוך אדידי. לשנה חזייה דהוה עציב, אמר ליה: אמאי עציבת? - אמר ליה: דלא אותיבי ערובי תבשילין. - אמר ליה: פושע את, לכולי עלמא - שרי, לדידך - אסור.

A certain blind man would recite *mishnayot* for Mar Shmuel, who saw that he was sad. He said to him, "Why are you sad?" He replied, "Because I did not prepare an *eruv tavshilin*." He told him, "rely on mine." Next year, he [again] saw that [the student] was sad. He said to him, "Why are you sad?" He replied, "Because I did not prepare an *eruv tavshilin*." He told him, "You are a sinner! Everyone else can [rely on me] but for you it is forbidden."

As Rashi explains, Mar Shmuel's *eruv tavshilin* was not meant to cover habitual sinners. This source implies that the blind are indeed obligated to keep the mitzvot. Nevertheless, it is understood that blindness may impair observance of certain mitzvot.[14]

Mishnah *Megillah* 4:6 (Bavli, 24a) addresses this point. After a general discussion of the qualifications for various synagogue rituals, the *Tanna Kamma* includes the blind in the category of Jews permitted to lead the ancient practice of *poreis al shema*:[15]

סוּמָא פּוֹרֵס אֶת שְׁמַע וּמְתַרְגֵּם. רַבִּי יְהוּדָה אוֹמֵר, כֹּל שֶׁלֹּא רָאָה מְאוֹרוֹת מִיָּמָיו, אֵינוֹ פּוֹרֵס עַל שְׁמַע:

The blind can be *poreis et shema* and can translate [the Torah into Aramaic as part of the reading]. Rabbi Yehudah says, whoever has never seen [the celestial] lights in his life[16] cannot be *poreis al shema*.[17]

Because of a significant textual variant of this Mishnah cited by the Rif, we will have cause to return to this text later. Meanwhile, Tosafot questions why Rabbi Yehudah needed to disqualify Jews who are blind from performing *this* specific mitzvah of פורס על שמע. Hadn't he already exempted them from "all mitzvot mentioned in the Torah"? Tosafot concludes that even Rabbi Yehudah considered blind Jews חייבין דרבנן– liable to keep all the commandments on the authority of the rabbis, lest they live like gentiles.[18] However, vision was an integral requirement to fulfill *poreis al shema*, and Rabbi Yehudah thus exempted them even from a rabbinic obligation for this mitzvah.

Although Jewish law followed the opinion of the Mishnah, namely that Jews who are blind are biblically commanded to keep the mitzvot,[19] Rabbi Yehudah's dissent continued to be influential. Rabbi Benjamin ben Mattathias explained that in disputes between Rabbi Meir and Rabbi Yehudah, the Halakha is usually according to Rabbi Yehudah.[20] The medieval scholar Rabbeinu Yerucham[21] cited the halakha that the blind are biblically exempt but nevertheless obligated to keep the mitzvot on rabbinic authority.[22] However, this point of view is explicitly rejected by later *poskim* such as Rabbi Yosef Karo[23] and the Radbaz.[24]

Thus far we have learned that a Jew who is blind has a general obligation to keep the mitzvot and may indeed lead the congregation in a variety of liturgical contexts. Mishnah Megillah 4:6 specifically allows blind Jews to serve as translator מתורגמן, which was an official role in the ancient Torah service. But can the סומא actually read Torah? As we shall see, there is a substantial literature addressing this question. One complication is that the terminology "read Torah" (יקרא בתורה) can refer to a number of activities, including chanting the Torah on behalf of the congregation, or reading the Torah blessings and listening as a reader chants from the Torah. It is not always obvious which sense the medieval halakhic sources intend.

THE OBLIGATION TO READ TORAH IN PUBLIC

Another complication is the status of Torah reading itself. Although many Jews assume that the public reading of the Torah is a biblical commandment, it is in fact a decree of the sages upon the community. Moses is traditionally credited with instituting the reading on Shabbat, Monday and Thursday, that Israel not go three days without Torah. Ezra instituted the reading on Shabbat afternoon as well as the accepted format.[25] Yet, as many *Rishonim*[26] and *Acharonim*[27] have written, this decree was made upon the congregation, and not upon each individual. The Torah blessings were added to honor the congregation, not to fulfill any specific obligation of the reader or the congregation.[28]

The lack of an individual obligation to read the Torah in public is alluded to by Ramban and Rambam and has been stated explicitly in recent responsa. For example, Rabbi Tzvi Pesach Frank, the twentieth century rabbi of Jerusalem known for his responsa *Har Tzvi,* writes:

שהקריאה היא רק חובת

הצבור שתקרא התורה בבית הכנסת, ואין צריך שיוציא הקורא רבים יד"ח

"for reading is an obligation only for the community that the Torah be read in synagogue, but the reader does not need to fulfill this obligation on behalf of the public."[29] It is presumably for this reason that the Tosefta allows Jews who are normally exempt from

מצות עשה שהזמן גרמא

to read Torah on behalf of the congregation.[30] This also would apparently qualify a Jew who is blind to read Torah, even according to Rabbi Yehudah. Thus the question is not whether a Jew who is blind is sufficiently obligated to fulfill this requirement on behalf of others. The question is whether the congregation's obligation can be satisfied with any method other than a direct reading from the Torah scroll.

THE PROHIBITION OF READING TORAH FROM MEMORY

The Rosh[31] concludes that the סומא is certainly obligated to obey the mitzvot, and can also fulfill mitzvot that bear rabbinic obligation such as *poreis al shema,* leading prayer, etc., on behalf of sighted individuals.[32] But at the end of his discussion, he adds one significant caveat:

הלכך אפילו לא ראה מאורות מימיו פורס על שמע ומתפלל, ובלבד שלא יקרא בתורה בעלפה.

Thus, even one who never in his life saw the lights can lead *poreis al shema* and pray [for the congregation], but he specifically must not read Torah from memory.

This *pesak* refers to the Talmudic maxim found on *Gitin* 60b,

דברים שבכתב אי אתה רשאי לאומרן על פה,

"words that are written must not be recited from memory."[33] This statement is applied by Maimonides to prohibit anyone from reading even one word of Torah or Megillah for the congregation from memory.[34]

The application of this prohibition to our case is stated already in the ninth century in the name of Rav Natronai Gaon:

מאור עינים...אינו קורא פרשת התורה מפני שאין העם יוצאים ידי חובתן ששומעים
בתורה מבעל פה, ואנו צריכים לשמוע מפי הקורא בכתב ולא בעל פה...ועל כן מאור
עיניים אע"פ שידע הפרשה ע"פ אסור לשמוע מפיו בבית הכנסת ואין יוצאים ידי חובה
שלא שמעו מן הכתב.

One who is blind may not chant the Torah portion because the people cannot fulfill their obligation by hearing the Torah [chanted] from memory but we need to hear from one reading the text, and not from memory. . . . Thus even if a blind person has memorized the portion, it is forbidden to hear him in synagogue, and the obligation [to chant Torah] is not fulfilled, for they have not heard [the Torah] from the text.[35]

This geonic edict, discussed by Rabbi Louis Ginzberg in *Geonica* (p. 121), clearly influenced many *Rishonim*, starting with the *Rosh*.

The *Rosh*'s conclusion excluding Jews who are blind from reading Torah "from memory" is codified by his son, Rabbi Jacob b. Asher. In his code, the *Arba'ah Turim,* two paragraphs reiterate this prohibition. At *Orach Chaim* 53, he restates his father's words:

סומא יכול לירד לפני התיבה ובלבד שלא יקרא בתורה שאין לקרות בתורה על פה:

The blind person may lead the congregation in prayer, but he specifically must not read the Torah, for one must not read Torah from memory.

At *Orach Chaim* 69, he reviews the ruling:

וכן כתב א"א ז"ל ש[סומא] יכול להתפלל ולהוציא אחרים ובלבד שלא יקרא בתורה
שאסור לקרות בעל פה:

And so too wrote my master, my father of blessed memory that [the blind] can pray and fulfill the obligations of others, but specifically must not read Torah [for others], for it is prohibited to read from memory.

Rabbi Yosef Karo then repeats this ruling in the *Beit Yosef* and *Shulchan Arukh*[36] at *Orach Chaim* 53:14. In the *Shulchan Arukh* to *Orach Chaim* 139:3, he rephrases the explanation for this restriction:

סומא אינו קורא, לפי שאסור לקרות אפי' אות אחת שלא מן הכתב.

The blind cannot read [Torah] for it is forbidden to read even one letter that is not from the written text.

Rabbi Karo's prohibition is well-grounded and conclusive.[37] Later authorities understood him to prohibit the blind *not only from reading Torah, but even from reciting the Torah blessings while a sighted reader chanted the text.*[38] The obstacle is not related to the obligations of the individuals, but to the status of the person who recites the Torah blessings (i.e., the *oleh*).

What would be the objection to the סומא reciting blessings while a sighted reader chanted from the scroll? The operative principle is

שומע כעונה,

the idea that a person may read Torah or Megillah vicariously by listening to an agent chant. In that way, the blessings s/he utters over the Torah are not considered לבטלה, in vain.

As Rabbi Norman Lamm and others show, there are two schools of thought regarding שומע כעונה, one narrow, and the other broad. The narrow school views the *oleh* as fully obligated to read along in the scroll, albeit with the assistance of a trained reader. The broad view is that the reader serves as an agent for the *oleh*, therefore obviating the need for the *oleh* to be capable, either intellectually or physically, of reading the actual Torah text. The former school, represented above, prohibits the blind not only from reading Torah, but even from having an *aliyah*, since the Torah blessings would then be said לבטלה, in vain.

Nevertheless, the halakha evolved in a more lenient direction based upon a broader application of שומע כעונה. Rabbi Isserles' gloss here adds a parenthetical clause:

(ומהרי"ל כתב דעכשיו קורא סומא, כמו שאנו מקרין בתורה לע"ה).

(But the Maharil[39] wrote that now we do read for the blind, just as we read the Torah for the unlettered.")

This gloss is the subject of substantial scholarly controversy. Rabbi Monique Susskind Goldberg shows in her paper that it is absent in the Cracow edition (1569-71), which was the first printing of the Shulchan Arukh together with the *Rema*.

Moreover, in *Darkhei Moshe,* his commentary to the *Beit Yosef,* Rabbi Isserles writes,

והמהרי"ל כתב דנוהגין לקרות סומא לס"ת ול"נ דברי הבית יוסף

"And the Maharil wrote that the custom is to call the blind up to the reading of the Torah, ול"נ the words of Beit Yosef." The crux is, of course, in the abbreviation ול"נ, which could stand either for ולי נראין "and I agree with," or ולא נראין "and [I] do *not* agree with" the *Beit Yosef*!

Rabbi Suskind Goldberg, following Rabbi Yaakov Emden, is convinced that Rabbi Isserles meant to accept the view of Rabbi Karo.[40] Yet Rabbi Lamm reads him the opposite way, and rejects the notion that Rabbi Isserles would have cited Maharil just in passing, even though he disagreed with his ruling.[41]

In any event, later *poskim* understood Rabbi Isserles as cited in the *Mapah,* namely, to reject Rabbi Karo's view, and to affirm the position of *Maharil* as recorded by his students in *Sefer Maharil,*[42]

אמר מהר"י סג"ל קורין לתורה אפי' עם הארץ. וכן הסומא, ולא נהגין כהרא"ש דפסק

דהסומא לא יקרא.

Moreinu HaRav Yaakov Sg"l[43] says that even the unlettered can be called [for an *aliyah*] to the Torah. And so too the blind, and we do not act in accordance with the Rosh, who ruled that the blind may not read.

The *Maharil* rejected the stricter practice of the *Rosh* (which was then cited by the *Tur* and *Shulchan Arukh*), who did not allow Jews who are blind even to recite the Torah blessings next to a designated reader.

A BROADER PRECEDENT?
THE CASE OF SEFER HAESHKOL

The *Maharil*'s permission has a precedent as early as Rabbi Abraham b. Isaac of Narbonne (1085-1158) in his *Sefer HaEshkol.*[44] This book is available in two printed editions, one edited in 1869 by Zevi Benjamin Auerbach (א.), and another version edited in 1935-8 by Shalom and Hanokh Albeck (ב.).[45] Because of significant variants between the two editions, I will present both of them, together with a version quoted by

Nimukei Yosef (ג.), although the latter may in fact be a paraphrase.[46] Addressing the question of whether a groom who is blind may be called to the Torah as is customary prior to the wedding, the *Eshkol* finds a leniency:

THE THREE EXTANT VERSIONS OF SEFER ESHKOL[47]

א Auerbach   **ב Albeck**   **ג** *Nimukei Yosef*

א. ותחן סומא א"א   למיתן לי'   תורה   דמעשה התול בעלמא הוא
ב. ותחן סומא לא אפשר למיתן ליה ספר תורה, דמעשה התול בעלמא הוא,
ג.

א. דהא   סומא לא יקרא בתורה[48]
ב. דתנן[49] סומא לא יקרא בתורה, והכי קאמ' לא יקרא על פה במקום מי שקורא
ג. אבל לא יקרא בתורה על פה במקום מי שקורא בתורה.

א.
ב. בכתב, דקיימ' לן דברים שבכתב אי אתה רשאי לאמרם על פה,
ג.

א. אבל אוקמי   אינש אחרינא   מברך ועומד בצדו ושפיר דמי.
ב. אבל לאוקמי אינש אחרינא[50] שפותח וראה ומברך ועומד מצדו, שפיר דמי.
ג. אבל אוקומי איניש אחרינא שפותח וראה והסומא מברך ועומד בצדו שפיר דמי

The following is my translation of the Albeck text, with the sections omitted by Auerbach marked in italic letters:

> It is not possible to give a blind groom the *Sefer* Torah [to read], for it is a disrespectful practice. For *it has been taught in a Mishnah that* the blind shall not read Torah. *But this means that he shall not read from memory in place of one who reads from the written text, for it has been established for us that things that are written may not be read from memory.* However, *to* bring up another man who *opens [the Sefer Torah] and sees,* blesses while he stands beside him, is a proper practice.

The Auerbach edition lacks the problematic reference to the "Mishnah" (see below) as well as the Eshkol's rationale for his suggestion. It also is more ambiguous about the mechanics of the proposed solution: "but to put another man up–he blesses and stands beside him–is considered proper." Who, precisely, does what?! The *Nimukei Yosef* mirrors elements of each Eshkol edition. However, he adds a crucial word at the end that clarifies that it is the blind man who utters the blessings and stands aside while his Torah portion is read from the text on his behalf.

The meaning of this text is rather opaque. In his commentary, Auerbach understands the *Eshkol* to mean that a sighted reader chants from the text, while the blind person reads the blessings and repeats the verses from memory (see note 48).

The Albeck edition seems to imply that it is the sighted man who stands to the side, reads the blessings and watches while the סומא chants the text. Yet in his commentary, Albeck cites the *Beit Yosef*'s rejection of *Eshkol*'s permission for a blind person to recite the blessings, and then adds,

ולפי הלשון כאן אפשר שגם למחברנו אין הסומא מברך אלא האחר וצ"ע,

"According to the wording here it is possible that, even according to our author, it is not the blind man who blesses, but the other [sighted person], and this needs inquiry" (see note 50). While this may mean that the blind person reads from memory, it may alternatively mean that the *Eshkol* allows the blind *neither* to read from the Torah *nor* to recite the blessings,[51] but simply to stand there, presumably in order to receive recognition as a groom. Yet this reading is difficult given *Nimukei Yosef*'s citation of *Eshkol*, and *Beit Yosef*'s criticism of his position as too permissive.

An additional issue posed by these variants is the Albeck edition's citation of a Mishnah that seems to prohibit the blind from "reading" Torah. Yet as we saw previously, the relevant Mishnah of Megillah 4:6 *does not* prohibit the blind from reading Torah. Where did the *Eshkol*'s citation come from? Albeck explains (note 49) that these words are indeed interpolated in the Rif's version of the Mishnah, as well as in an early "*Yilamdeinu*" Midrash in *Tanchuma* Toldot 7:7 as follows:

ילמדנו רבינו סומא מהו שיעבור לפני התיבה להוציא את הצבור,
כך שנו רבותינו סומא פורס על שמע ומתרגם, אבל אינו עובר לפני התיבה
ואינו קורא בתורה ואינו נושא את כפיו.

These versions of the Mishnah prohibit Jews who are blind not only from reading Torah, but also from leading the congregation in prayer and reciting the priestly benediction.

If, in fact, the Mishnah had explicitly prohibited calling blind Jews to the Torah, this entire discussion might not have developed. Yet Rabbi Susskind Goldberg shows that this textual variant shows up in *none* of the extant manuscripts of the Mishnah or of the Talmud itself. The *Bah* already noted that this text was lacking in the gemara, in *Piskei HaRosh*, and in *Alfasi Yashan*. Indeed, *Dikdukei Sofrim* argues that these words were a later corruption of the Rif's text.[52]

Whether or not the Mishnah had actually prohibited the blind from reading Torah, *Sefer HaEshkol* clearly identifies the probable objection–that he not recite the text from memory on behalf of the congregation.

The *Eshkol* is cited approvingly by *Nimukei Yosef,* although he indicates that he did not have the original text before him. There remains significant confusion about the meaning of *Eshkol*'s words. Did he really imply that the blind could read from memory so long as a sighted reader followed along? Quietly, or audibly? The *Nimukei Yosef* and then *Beit Yosef* understood him (as did Auerbach) to justify only calling blind Jews up to bless the Torah while the reader chanted on their behalf. This seems to be the most defensible reading of Sefer Eshkol.

The fourteenth century *Sefer HaAgudah*,[53] cited by *Beit Yosef* in connection to the *Eshkol*, dismisses the various objections to calling a סומא who is a Kohen up for an *aliyah*:

ונראה לי במקום דליכא כהן בעיר אלא סומא, נראה דמותר לקרותו לס"ת ולא יאמר אין
כאן כהן, כיון דקריאת התורה מדרבנן יכול הסומא להוציאם, ואי משום ברכה לבטלה
הלא גם הרואה פטור מלברך דהא בירך שחרית, אלא שמחייב את עצמו, הכי נמי לא
שנא, ואי משום דברים שבכתב אי אתה רשאי לאומרם בע"פ לא, דבזה"ז אינו קורא אלא
החזן.

It seems to me that in a place where there is no Kohen in the city other than a blind one, that it is permitted to call him to the Torah. They must not say, "there is no Kohen here" for reading the Torah is a rabbinic obligation and a blind Jew can discharge it for them. And if [one objects that his would be] a blessing in vain, aren't even the sighted exempt from blessing since they have already [blessed the Torah] in the Shacharit [service]? Rather [the *oleh*] obligates himself, and so too in this case it is no different. And if [one objects] that words which are written must not be said from memory, this is not a problem, for in our time, he does not actually read, but rather, it is the *hazzan*.[54]

Yet again, the most vigorous defense of a blind Jew participating in the Torah service is an affirmation that he may have an *aliyah*.

דברי האחרונים *EARLY MODERN PRACTICE*

The *Taz*[55] decides in favor of calling Jews who are blind up for an *aliyah*–even if they are not learned:[56]

וכתוב בלבוש שראה בפני גדולים שעלה סומא לתורה וכ"כ מו"ח ז"ל רק שהתנה שצריך
שיהיה הסומא ת"ח ולא ע"ה ומצד ההוכחה נלע"ד גם כן היתר גמור.

It is written in the *Levush*[57] that he observed [an incident] in the presence of great sages that a blind man was called up to the Torah [for an *aliyah*]. And so too wrote my teacher and father-in-law[58] of blessed memory. Yet he stipulated that the blind man must be a scholar, and not unlettered. Based on the proof offered, it seems in my humble opinion to be completely permissible.

The *Taz*'s ruling was adopted as Ashkenazi practice, as seen in the *Mishnah Berurah* to *Orach Chaim* 139:12-13, who further clarifies the rationale for calling a Jew who is blind up to recite the Torah blessings:

(יב) ... דעכשיו קורא סומא -וטעמו דכיון שאנו נוהגין שהש"ץ קורא והוא קורא מתוך
הכתב שוב לא קפדינן על העולה דשומע כעונה:

(12) . . . For now the blind are called up, and the reason is that because we have a reader who reads from the written text we are no longer strict about the *oleh* [literally reading from the text], for hearing is like answering.

(יג) כמו שאנו וכו' - ר"ל שאנו נוהגין להקל אפילו אם אינו יכול לקרות עם הש"ץ מלה
במלה מתוך הכתב וע"כ מטעם הנ"ל וה"ה בסומא. ולדינא כבר כתבו האחרונים דנהגו
להקל כמהרי"ל ומ"מ לפרשת פרה ופרשת זכור נכון שלא לקרותן לכתחלה:

(13) "As we etc." That is to say, that we act leniently [allowing an unlettered person his *aliyah*] even if he cannot read with the reader word for word from the written text, and this is surely for the above mentioned reason, and is also the rule for the blind. And in practice, the *Acharonim* have already written to act leniently according to the Maharil. However, it is proper not to call them up for *Parshat Parah* and *Parshat Zachor ab initio*.

As we have seen, the *Mishnah Berurah* follows the *Taz* in understanding the principle of דשומע כעונה (that listening is like responding) in the broad sense, thereby allowing a Jew who is either physically or intellectually (or both) unable to read Torah to have an *aliyah* and listen to the reader. At 49:1:2, the *Mishnah Berurah* explains that a blind person may in fact read Torah from memory *for himself*; it is only the act of reading from memory in order to fulfill the obligations of *others* that is prohibited.[59]

The established custom is therefore that Jews who are blind may not read from memory to fulfill the congregation's mandate. Rather, they are honored with *aliyot* to the Torah to recite the blessings and to have their portion read on their behalf, and may certainly repeat the text softly.

The stringent perspective reflected in the Rosh, Tur and by Rabbi Karo is forcefully restated by the eighteenth century Rabbi Jacob b. Tzvi Emden[60] in his responsa, שאילת יעבץ.[61] Emden rejects the notion that a Jew who is blind can even recite the Torah blessings and respond to the sighted reader in the manner that sighted Jews do:

> דקמשמע לן דסומא לא יקרא כלל, ואפי' ע"י שישמע מאחר, המקרא אותו בלחש והוא
> עונה אחריו, דפקח כח"ג מצי עביד גם לפי מנהג התלמוד, וכמנהג בני רומני שהובא בב"י.
>
> ... This teaches us that the blind may not read [Torah] at all, even via hearing from another who dictates to him quietly so that he can repeat afterwards, for [only] a sighted person in such circumstances can follow the custom of the Talmud, and of the Romaniot Jews as cited in the *Beit Yosef.*

Rabbi Emden rejects the broad interpretation of שומע כעונה, and he goes so far as to question whether the Maharil really supported this custom, or merely acquiesced to a popular practice that was objectionable. However, Emden admits that he did not have a copy of the Maharil's work before him.[62] As we have seen, Maharil states his opinion quite clearly, and later authorities such as the *Mishnah Berurah* reaffirm the legitimacy of this practice. As noted above, Rabbi Emden doubts whether Rabbi Isserles had indeed endorsed the Maharil's view, but the available evidence suggests otherwise. The other *Rishonim* cited by Emden oppose allowing the blind to read Torah from memory, but do not explicitly reject their reciting the Torah blessings and listening to a sighted reader chant from the Torah.

The stringent opinion of Rabbi Emden is rejected by the contemporary *poseik* Rabbi Ovadiah Yosef in a responsum dealing initially with whether the Torah blessings must be recited when transcribing the Torah.[63] In the course of that discussion, he quotes the view of the Radbaz to the effect that if one looked at a word in the text of the Torah and then lifted his eyes but said the word immediately, it is considered as having actually read the word. Then he seeks support for this view by quoting the *Sefer HaEshkol,* who permits a blind Jew to recite the Torah blessings, and he says:

והרי מבואר בב"י שם עפ"ד הרא"ש והטור שחייב העולה לקרות בס"ת בנחת אחר הש"ץ
דאי לא"ה הו"ל ברכה לבטלה. וא"כ כיון שאין הש"ץ מוציאו, והסומא אינו רואה הקריאה
כלל, מה תועלת בראיית הש"ץ הכתב בס"ת הרי צריך העולה לס"ת לקרות ממש מתוך
הכתב. א"ו שמכיון שהש"ץ רואה וקורא מתוך הכתב, והסומא קורא אחריו בנחת בתכ"ד
לראייתו של הש"ץ שפיר דמי. אלמא דלא בעינן שהקריאה של העולה לס"ת תהיה מתוך
הכתב ממש.

It is explained in *Beit Yosef* (ibid.) based upon the *Rosh* and the *Tur* that the *oleh* is obligated to read in the Torah scroll quietly after the designated reader, for if not for this, his would be a wasted blessing. If so, since the designated reader does not fulfill the [*oleh*'s] obligations vicariously, and the blind [*oleh*] doesn't see the text at all, what benefit is there that the reader sees the text [for him] in the Torah scroll? Doesn't the *oleh* to the Torah need truly to read from the text? Rather it must be the case that when the reader sees and reads from the text, and the blind [*oleh*] repeats after him quietly without any delay from the reader, that this is considered proper. *Infer that we do not require that the reading of the oleh to the Torah be literally from the text.*

Thus, claims Rabbi Yosef, the Eshkol's permission to grant an *aliyah* to a blind person can be explained only if one understands the Radbaz as explained above.[64]

There are two schools of thought about the principle of שומע כעונה, and thus the role of the בעל קורא, the designated Torah reader; these correspond to the two schools which we have identified regarding the blind receiving an *aliyah* to the Torah. According to Rabbi Emden, the designated reader does *not* fulfill the *oleh*'s obligations on his behalf. Rather the *oleh* must read for himself at the same time that the designated reader chants aloud to the congregation. In Rabbi Emden's view, this precludes a blind Jew from reciting the Torah blessings; because he cannot read the Torah text, his blessings are in vain.

Rabbi Yosef considers this approach, but rejects it based on the established precedents of *Maharil, Rema* and the *Taz* allowing blind Jews to be called for *aliyot*. For him, the sighted designated reader does indeed vicariously fulfill the obligation of the *oleh* to read the Torah text after reciting the blessings. Rabbi Yosef's son Yitzhak, writing in

Yalkut Yosef, confirms this practice of calling the blind up for *aliyot,* although he prefers that they be granted only additional *aliyot* or *maftir.* Nevertheless, if the blind person is a Kohen, he may be called up for the first *aliyah,* so long as the reader chants the text, and the *oleh* repeats quietly after him.[65] In his notes, *Yalkut Yosef* cites the responsum of Rabbi Eliezer Waldenburg, who records that the practice among all Ashkenazim (based on the *Rema*) and most Sephardim is to call the blind up for an *aliyah.*[66] He further criticizes an authority who embarrassed a blind Jew by refusing to allow him an *aliyah.*[67]

A new book called ספר הסומא, by Rabbi Aryeh Rodriguez lists dozens of halakhic sources, ancient to contemporary, on both sides of this debate. By now, the prevalent custom in Israel (with the possible exception of Safed, in deference to Rabbi Karo) and the diaspora is to call Jews who are blind up for *aliyot* to the Torah.[68] Is it possible to add one more level of participation so that Jews who are blind might somehow chant not only the Torah blessings, but also the Torah text? This is the question posed to us by Rabbi Krishef.

THE SEARCH FOR AN EXPANDED ROLE FOR THE BLIND

Three halakhic obstacles lie in the path of Jews who are blind and who wish to read Torah. As we have learned, the first obstacle is the status of their obligation. Had the law followed Rabbi Yehudah and then Rabbeinu Yerucham, Jews who are blind might have been disqualified even from receiving an *aliyah* to the Torah based on their exemption from the mitzvah of Torah study. However, the law instead obligated blind Jews to observe the mitzvot in general. Moreover, we have seen that there is not truly an individual obligation for the Torah reading, and that even individuals who are exempt from Torah study can serve as agents of the congregation by chanting Torah.

The second obstacle is the prohibition of reading "even one letter of a written text from memory." This Talmudic maxim is cited by all medieval authorities on our subject, as noted above. Clearly, this rules out the first suggestion of the שאלה. But since the development of a Hebrew braille system in the 1930s and the printing of braille Chumashim, and the more recent advances in optical scanning, the objection that blind Jews would have to rely on memory in order to chant Torah has been removed. *The specific objections raised in the codes of the Rosh and his followers are nullified when the Jew who is blind reads from a braille Chumash.*

Nevertheless, there remains a third obstacle which is not so easily cleared. The congregation's obligation to hear the Torah read is fulfilled only via a kosher Torah scroll, not from a printed book. Rabbi Moshe Isserles writes (*Orach Chaim* 143:2),

אבל בחומשים שלנו אפילו כל ה' ספרים ביחד אין לברך עליהם.

But as for our [printed] Pentateuchs–even if all five books are included–we do not recite the [Torah] blessings over them.

The *Mishnah Berurah* here (143:2:9) adds that if, lacking a Sefer Torah, the congregation uses a printed Chumash (שלא תשתכח תורת קריאה "lest the skill of reading Torah be forgotten"), congregants are not called up for *aliyot*, but the reader simply recites the text aloud for the congregation.

Interestingly, the *Mishnah Berurah* cites another custom (143:2:10) for congregations that do own a Sefer Torah, but lack a reader qualified to chant from the scroll:

והאידנא נהגים שאחד קורא מהחומש בלחש והש"ץ קורא אחריו מס"ת משום דיש אנשים שאין יודעין לקרות בניגון וטעמים ואפילו מקרין אותם לכן מקרין לש"ץ.

The current practice is for one to read softly from the Chumash and the reader repeats after him from the Sefer Torah, for there are people who do not know how to read with the melody and cantillation, even if we dictate to them; thus we also dictate to the reader.

The congregation's obligation to read the Torah at its prescribed time is met only when a reader chants from a kosher Torah scroll. This presumably would exclude Jews who are blind from chanting from a braille edition of the Chumash in order to fulfill the obligations of the congregation. *A braille Chumash, like any printed Chumash, may be used as a guide, but not as a substitute for a kosher Sefer Torah.*

Although Jews who are blind may receive *aliyot* to the Torah, there is no established mechanism for them to read the Torah itself for the congregation. On the other hand, it is permissible for the blind to read Haftarah–which does not require a hand-written scroll–on behalf of the congregation. This ruling is made explicit in a responsum of *Minchat Yitzhak*.[69]

Thus a Jew who is blind may certainly lead services, recite the Torah and Haftarah blessings, and chant Haftarah, whether for a Bar/Bat Mitzvah celebration or in the normal course of services.[70] Nevertheless, learning to read Torah is a powerful and important task in the Jewish life cycle. It symbolizes קבלת עול תורה, acceptance of the Torah as a reenactment of the revelation at Mount Sinai. For many centuries Jews have linked their celebrations as well as their solemn commemoration of *yahrzeit* with the reading of Torah. Is there any method for including the blind in this sacred act?

POSSIBLE PATHS AROUND THE STUMBLING BLOCK

Rabbi Krishef has asked whether a scanning device could be used by a Jew who is blind to read Torah, much as visually impaired Jews read via spectacles. In fact, such a machine, called the Optacon, does exist, although it is no longer manufactured. Dr. Abraham Nemeth, a highly proficient reader, demonstrated the use of this machine for me. It replicates on a vibrating touch pad the shape of any images captured by photoelectric cells at the tip of a wand. When the wand is placed against a white surface, there is no response, but when it encounters print, it causes the touch pad to vibrate in the same pattern. This device could allow a Jew who is blind to feel the actual text of the Torah scroll without any intervening optical character recognition (OCR) technology. S/he would literally read מן הכתב "from the writing." Unfortunately, the Optacon is an obsolete device, and is noisy and very unwieldy, even for an expert. It would not be possible to use it to read at normal speeds since it takes a moment to find and identify each letter. Use of such technology on Shabbat and Yom Tov would introduce new complications such as writing.

Nevertheless, should technology improve to the point that the actual Torah scroll could be read by blind Jews, even as visually impaired Jews read the Torah using corrective devices today, we may have an ideal solution, at least for weekdays. Further study of the developing technology is required.[71] People who are not fully blind may certainly use magnifying devices in order to read Torah.

Another theoretical possibility would be to add braille text between the lines of a Sefer Torah. Yet this is problematic. Vocalized Torah (codex) scrolls are not used for congregational reading of Torah, and the braille would not fit between the lines or columns. Indeed, the Torah scroll would have to be enormous given the need for additional space and the fact that braille marks would prevent the scroll from being wrapped as tightly as is customary. Lastly, the reader would not benefit from the visible ink of the scroll and thus the written text would not itself be read. The Talmud's dictate remains that scripture be read

מן הכתב,
from the actual text.

A better alternative is to distinguish the *maftir* reading from the rest of the *parashah*. Already in the Gemara (*Megillah* 23a), the *maftir's* reading of Torah is set apart from the rest of the portion. His status as one of the mandatory seven Shabbat readers is subject to debate. According to Ulla, his repetition of a passage of Torah prior to chanting the Haftarah is simply out of deference for the Torah, rather than fulfillment of a communal obligation.

In contrast, Tosafot cites the halakha according to the opinion that the *maftir's* Torah reading *does* count fully. This position is supported by normative practice on occasions such as fast day afternoons in which the third reader also serves as *maftir*. Moreover, on days such as Rosh Hodesh, festivals, Shabbat Parah and Shabbat Zakhor in which the *maftir* reads a special section for חובת היום–the required daily theme– he is certainly fulfilling the congregation's obligation through his Torah reading. In such cases, the Torah must be read directly from the scroll.

Nonetheless, on a regular Shabbat, the *maftir's* reading of Torah is not in fulfillment of any public obligation. As Rambam notes, the reader's kaddish between the end of the portion and the *maftir* separates him from the seven mandatory readers.[72] This ruling is confirmed by Rabbi Isserles.[73] We have seen that the barrier to reading from memory is specific to cases in which the reader is fulfilling the obligation of others.[74] If so, then a Jew who is blind could read the *maftir* Torah section from a braille Chumash, since this is neither prohibited as a recitation from memory, nor insufficient to fulfill a public obligation which does not truly exist.

Given what we have learned, there are three practical options for a Jew who is blind to participate in קריאת התורה, the chanting of the Torah:

1. שומע ועונה. When called up for his *aliyah*, the Jew who is blind listens to the chanting and ideally follows in a braille Chumash. After each word or phrase, the reader pauses and allows the blind *oleh* softly to repeat the text. This solution has ample precedent,[75] but it would possibly be least satisfying to the *oleh* and to the congregation.

2. עולה ומתרגם. Mishnah Megillah 4:3 specifically permits a Jew who is blind to serve as translator, a role which involved interpolating Aramaic translation between *each* Hebrew verse.[76] Indeed,

the blind Rav Yosef was considered an expert in this task.[77] Although this custom has fallen into disuse (with the notable exception of the Yemenite rite), it remains a perfectly valid option.[78] The blind reader can perform an important service for the congregation by translating the Torah into the common language as it is read from the scroll, verse by verse. If done for the entire portion, this might become an imposition, but it could be used as a teaching tool for a specific selection. Indeed, there has been recent movement to reinstitute the ritual translation of Torah as a dramatic and effective educational tool.

3. חוזר וקורא. A third option is for the congregation to complete its reading of the *parashah*, and then to call the Jew who is blind to repeat the *maftir* or even a longer passage from a braille text. The Torah blessings would be said while holding onto the *atzei chaim* of the scroll as a way of giving כבוד לתורה, honor to the Torah, and to address the concerns of Rabbi Isserles cited previously. If the blind reader is not also saying the blessings, and the *oleh* is sighted, then he or she should follow in the scroll.

The third adaptation could not be practiced on days when *maftir* is read from a second scroll, but would not pose a problem on regular Shabbatot. The congregation would have already discharged its obligation to have the *parashah* chanted in the established format from the Torah scroll. The blind reader would obligate him or herself for the additional reading and blessings. His/her act of blessing the Torah and chanting its words would certainly be a public sanctification of God's name.

CONCLUSION

Jews who are blind should participate in synagogue rituals together with sighted Jews, all of whom are obligated to keep the Torah. Indeed, it is in the interest of the Jewish community to include as many Jews as possible in the rituals of studying Torah and fulfilling mitzvot. As we have seen, Jews who are blind may:

a. Lead the congregation in prayer;
b. Receive an *aliyah* and chant the appropriate blessings;
c. Chant *haftarah*.

Because the Torah must be read for the congregation directly from a Torah scroll, and not from a printed text or from memory, Jews who are blind may participate in Torah reading in one of three ways:

a. By receiving an *aliyah* and chanting softly after the reader;
b. By serving as *meturgamon*, the verse-by-verse translator of a section of the *parashah*;
c. By reading from braille a standard *maftir,* since it has already been chanted in the established fashion from the Sefer Torah.

Should new technology that allows blind people to read directly from the scroll become available, our options would expand. Meanwhile, these solutions all preserve our reverence for the sacred act of chanting Torah from a kosher scroll, while also allowing Jews who are blind to be included in the act of publicly accepting and revering the Torah.

כך נלע"ד

והערב נא ה' אלקינו את דברי תורתך בפינו ובפי עמך בית ישראל.
May the words of Your Torah, Adonai our God, be sweet in our mouths and in the mouths of Your people, the household of Israel.

NOTES

1. I thank Rabbi David Krishef for the initial inquiry and sources for this responsum.

2. I am grateful for the advice on this topic of Professor Abraham Nemeth, a remarkable member of my congregation who is the creator of the "Nemeth Code" for marking mathematical notation in braille. See his article in *Braille into the Next Millennium* (Washington, D.C.: National Library for the Blind and Physically Handicapped, 2000). I have also benefited from the advice of Rabbi Michael Levy, who is a board member of the Jewish Braille Institute of America. His article, "To Stand on Holy Ground: A Jewish Spiritual Perspective on Disability" (*Rehabilitation Education,* Volume 9, No. 2 and 3, 1995, pp. 163-170) deepened my understanding of the integration of physical disability into the mission of serving God with one's life. Rabbis Joel Roth, Mayer Rabinowitz and David Fine were all very helpful in locating obscure sources and reviewing this *teshuvah* with me.

3. Late in this project I found four excellent overviews on the blind and halakha: Dr. Avraham Steinberg, (תחומין ג' תשמ"ב) העיור בהשקפת היהדות, Rabbi Norman Lamm, (תורה שבעל פה, לא, תש"ן) חיוב סומא במצוות, Rabbi Monique Susskind Goldberg, העיוור בהלכה, עיון בכמה שאלות הלכתיות (unpublished Masters/Ordination thesis, Machon Schechter, 1999) and Rabbi Aryeh Rodriguez, (ירושלים: בית חנוך מורים תשס"ב) ספר סומא.

There is also a Hasidic overview by Rabbi David H. Toiv, Director of the Jewish Heritage for the Blind, entitled *Halakhic Rulings Relating to the Blind* (NY: The Jewish Heritage for the Blind, 1997). These articles are cited below.

4. This is established in the prior discussion on B.K. 86a and is then reflected in the commentaries of Rashi and Tosafot. See next note.

5. רש"י ב"ק פו ע"ב ד"ה דלא כרבי יהודה. דאמר סומא אין לו בושת אם בייש חבירו פטור ומתניתין קתני ישן שבייש פטור ובסומא לא תנא הכי הלכך סומא חייב.

6. That is, the anonymous voice of the Mishnah. On B.K. 86a the source of this teaching is ultimately attributed to Rabbi Shimon, though some *Rishonim* identify this view with Rabbi Meir.

7. תוספות שם, ד"ה סומא.

8. בבא קמא פז ע"א, ובמקביל בשינוים קטנים בקדושין לא ע"א.

9. שמות פרק יג, פסוק ח. והגדת לבנך ביום ההוא לאמר בעבור זה עשה ה' לי בצאתי ממצרים:

10. בננו זה. This גזירה שוה depends on the assumption that the parents' statement to the elders was accompanied by a visual identification of their son. See Rashi,

ד"ה פרט לסומין.

11. This story can be harmonized with Rabbi Yehudah's position based on the claim that the mitzvah of Hagadda is rabbinic, and Rabbi Yehudah agrees that blind Jews share general rabbinic obligations. See below, note 18.

12. Rabbi Israel Francus cited this text in his article published in *The Ordination of Women as Rabbis* (NY: JTSA, 1988, p. 38) as proof that a person who is obligated rabbinically cannot upgrade to a biblical obligation. Yet Rabbi Joel Roth, writing in the same volume, argues that the self-imposed obligation of women to observe mitzvot from which they were traditionally exempted is indeed legally significant (see esp. pp. 141-148). In any event, the halakha for blind Jews ultimately follows the *stam mishnah* and fully obligates them to observe the commandments.

13. *Eruv tavshilin.* This is a symbolic amount of food set aside before a festival begins which allows food to be prepared during the festival for the Shabbat which immediately follows. It is customary to state one's intention that others be covered by the *eruv tavshilin* in case they forgot to prepare one themselves.

14. One example is קרבן ראיה, the "appearance" offering presented by pilgrims in Jerusalem at the three festivals. See note 24 below and the Steinberg article for other examples.

15. The custom of collectively reciting the blessings before the Shema, especially ברכת יוצר, which praises God for creating the celestial lights. See Rashi on Sotah 30b: כסופר. מתחיל בברכות שלפני קריאת שמע והן. See also S.A. O.H. 69:1.

עונין אחריו וקורין כולן יחד וכך שרתה רוח הקודש על כולם וכוונו יחד את השירה ככתבה.

16. This leads to a theoretical discussion in the Yerushalmi, and then the Rosh and Tosafot, about whether the disqualification requires that the person be truly blind, or whether a person raised in a cave who simply had never seen the sun and moon could recite these blessings for the congregation.

17. One version of this Mishnah, which is cited by the Rif (p. 15a) and in one variant of *Sefer HaEshkol,* adds the words אבל אינו קורא בתורה, "but he must not read Torah." See below, p. 11.

18. בבא קמא פז ע"א ד"ה וכן (ג). ותע"ע בתוספות מסכת ראש השנה לג ע"א ד"ה הא רבי יהודה הא רבי יוסי "...שלא יראה כנכרי דאם פטור ליה בכל מצות נמצא דאינו נוהג בתורת ישראל כלל."

19. בית יוסף או"ח סוף ס' תעג, ובמשנה ברורה ס' נג ס"ק מא.

20. Rabbi Benjamin ben Mattatias, Greece and Venice, early sixteenth century, writing in his responsa,

שו"ת בנימין זאב סימן רמה ד"ה וכן מצאתי.

He concludes, nevertheless, based on the Bava Kama text and its subsequent interpretation that, even according to Rabbi Yehudah, the blind are obligated to read and bless the Torah.

21. Provençe and Spain, 1280-1350.

22. רבינו ירוחם - תולדות אדם נתיב יג חלק א דף קג טור א "סומא פטור מכל המצות. פירוש מדאוריתא אבל מדרבנן חייב כך פשוט בקדושין וכן מוכח בפסחים דחייב מדרבנן וכן מוכח שם דמוציא אחרים בדבר שחייבין מדרבנן ורבינו תם כתב שמברך על המצות שפטור עליו ויש חולקין עליו ומחלקתם כתבתי נתיב כ"ז ח"א בעניין נשים כי דינם שוה."

Rabbeinu Yerucham writes: "The blind are exempt from all mitzvot. This means biblically exempt, but rabbinically obligated. This is clear in *Kiddushin* and also found in *Pesahim* that he is rabinically obligated—thus it is proven in that he fulfills the rabbinic obligations of others. And Rabbeinu Tam wrote that one can recite the blessing over mitzvot from which s/he is exempt. But others disagree with him as I have written in section 27, part 1 regarding women, for their status is identical (to the blind)."

23. בית יוסף אורח חיים סימן תעג ד"ה המוזגין מיד. "ולית הלכתא כוותיה [כר"י] ומיהו מה שכתב דמכל מקום חייב בכל מדרבנן כ"כ התוספות בפרק החובל (ד"ה וכן דבור שני) אליבא דרבי יהודה" ובאורח חיים סימן נג אות יד ד"ה סומא יכול כתב "דסומא חייב בכל המצות."

Beit Yosef writes, "The law is not like him [i.e., Rabbi Yehudah]. Yet he wrote that in any event, [the blind] are obligated by the Rabbis, and so too wrote Tosafot in *Perek HaHoveil* based upon Rabbi Yehudah." B.Y. writes further, "For the blind are obligated in all the mitzvot."

24. Rabbi David b. Solomon ibn Avi Zimra (1479-1573). He writes in a responsum, Section I, number 39,

ד"ה תשובה לכאורת. "...וכבר הוכחתי כן בתשובה אחרת מהתלמוד ומדברי כל הפוסקים ולא מצאתי לרבינו ירוחם ז"ל חבר בסברא זו דאין הלכה כר' יהודה אלא כסתמא דמתני' דסומא הרי הוא כאדם בריא לכל דברי חוץ מלענין עדות והגדה וסנהדרין ומלקרוא בתורה לפי שהוא כקורא על פה ועליהם לרגל וחגיגה ומכל אלה נתמעט הסומא בהדיא ומינה אתה למד דלכל שאר הדברים הרי הוא כאדם שלם וחייב בכל מצות האמורות בתורה."

"And I have already proven this (in another responsum) from the Talmud and the words of all the *poskim*, and I have not found a companion for Rabbeinu Yerucham z"l in his opinion [exempting the blind], for the law is not according to R. Yehudah, but rather according to the *stamma* of our Mishnah that the blind man is like a healthy person in all regards with the exception of testimony, Haggadah, [serving in] the Sanhedrin, and reading Torah because it is like reading from memory [see below, p. 7], and the pilgrimage and the festive offering. For all of these the blind man is explicitly excluded. From this you learn that in other matters he is like a whole [healthy] individual, and is obligated by all the mitzvot in the Torah."

25. בבא קמא פב ע"א. ברמב"ם הלכות תפילה פרק יב, הל' א.

26. Following Ramban in *Milchamot Hashem* to RIF, *Megillah* p. 3. For an excellent discussion of the nature of the obligation to chant Torah, see R. Mendel Shapiro's article "Qeri'at ha-Torah by Women: A Halakhic Analysis" in *The Edah Journal* 1:2 (Sivan 5761), p. 5f. He observes that this distinction is also implicit in Rambam, who places the rules of Torah reading apart from the individual prayers and just after the laws of synagogues. The Shapiro article and several related pieces are available on-line at www.edah.org.

27. עיין לדוגמה בשו"ת יביע אומר חלק ח-או"ח סימן יד ד"ה ד) "ומדברי: ...מה שאין כן קריאת התורה שחחיוב רק שישמע קריאת התורה. וחכמים תיקנו לברך משום כבוד הצבור וכו'. ואילו מדברי הרמב"ן והר"ן מוכח שגם עיקר קריאת התורה אינה אלא חובת צבור." וע"ע בשו"ת אגרות משה חלק א"ח א' סימן כח ד"ה ויש חלוק: "לענין קריאת התורה דבזה לכ"ע הוא חובת הצבור." ובשו"ת ציץ אליעזר ח"ז סי' א-קונטרס קטן למפטיר פרק ה ד"ה אולם בשו"ת: "לפי שהל' קריאה היא חובת הצבור."

28. Other explanations for the Torah blessings include to honor the Torah, as well as a קל וחמר from food, which requires blessings before and after. How much more so does the spiritual sustenance of Torah study require blessings! See ד"ה ובעשיית המצות ספר אבודרהם, ברכת המצות ומשפטיהם.

29. שו"ת הר צבי או"ח א סימן עב ד"ה ומה שדן.

30. תוספתא מגילה פ"ג הלכה יא.

31. Rabbeinu Asher b. Yechiel, 1250-1327, Germany and Spain.

32. שו"ת הרא"ש כלל ד סימן כא, וע"ע בכלל ג סימן יב.

33. ועיין לגבי מקרא מגילה בתוספתא מגילה פרק ב הלכה ה, "קראה על פה לא יצא ידי חובתו" ובירושלמי מגילה כח ע"ב.

34. רמב"ם הלכות תפילה ונשיאת כפים פרק יב הלכה ת. "והוא שלא יקרא על פה שאסור לקרות שלא מן הכתב אפילו תיבה אחת"

35. שערי תשובה ס' רמת. ראה בייסקינד גולדברג, ע' 32.

36. סומא יורד לפני התיבה, ובלבד שלא יקרא בתורה, משום: דברים שבכתב אי אתה רשאי לאומרם על פה.

37. Especially *Beit Yosef* to O.H. 141:2 ד"ה ומ"ש where Rabbi Karo cites numerous authorities and explicitly rejects the lenient position of the *Eshkol* (see below) and of his followers.

38. See below, p. 13.

39. Moreinu Jacob b. Moses HaLevi Moellin, Germany and Austria, 1360-1427. Ed. Shlomo Spitzer, Jerusalem, 5749.

40. העיוור בהלכה, עיון בכמה שאלות הלכתיות, ע' 34. "מכאן ברור שהרמ"א תנצגד לעליית העיוור לתורה."

41. נחום לאם, "חיוב סומא בהלכה" תורה שבעל פה, לא, תש"ן עמ' קו-קק, הערה 2. "ובדקתי בכל הוצאות הד"מ שיצאו לאור לפני זמנו של הרי"ע וגם בזמנו, עד כדי שידי מגעת, ובעיקר משנת תקכ"ב שמסתבר ביותר שהיא ההוצאה של דרכי משה שהגרי"ע השתמש בו, ובכולן מובא כדברים שהזכרנו. ייתכן שהרי"ע פירש ראשי התיבות "ולי"נ" כ"ולי נראין" ואילו הרמ"א באמת התכוון לומר "ולא נראין".

42. ספר מהרי"ל (מנהגים) הלכות קריאת התורה ד"ה [ג] נשאל.

43. That is, "our teacher Jacob, סגן לכהן, assistant to the priest," i.e. a Levite.

44. ספר האשכול (אלבק) הלכות קריאת התורה, ע' 184, דף סח עמוד ב. ובמהדורת אוערבך, ע' 69.

45. It is worth citing Saul Aaron Adler's article in the *Encyclopedia Judaica*, s.v. Abraham ben Isaac of Narbonne: "The *Eshkol* was first published by Zevi Benjamin Auerbach (1869) with an introduction and commentary, but doubts about the authenticity of at least parts of Auerbach's manuscript were expressed by Shalom Albeck. The ensuing controversy was inconclusive. Auerbach's manuscript is rich in additions, the exact origin of which is not clear. Although there are no grounds for accusing Auerbach of willfully tampering with the manuscript, the version of the *Eshkol* that Albeck had in hand is undoubtedly the authentic one. Albeck himself published part of the *Sefer ha-Eshkol* (with introductions and notes) and his son Hanokh Albeck completed this edition (1935-38)."

46. Rabbi Joseph Habiba, early 15th century Spain. *Nimukei Yosef* to *Megillah* is not included in its usual place around the Rif. In 1960 (5720) Moshe Blau published an edition of the *Nimukei Yosef* to *Megillah* and *Pesachim*. He quotes the *Eshkol* [misidentified as ספר השכול], but apparently indirectly:

ויש מי שכתב מספר השכול....

This version of the text of *Nimukei Yosef* is also quoted in *Beit Yosef* (O.H. 141:2).

47. ספר האשכול, הלכות סדר פרשיות והפטרות לכל שוי"ט ולתעניות, חלק א.

48. Auerbach explains Eshkol's rationale for allowing the blind an *aliyah*:

לג' רי"ף כ"כ במש', ונסחתו מגילה כ"ד סומא פורס על שמע ומתרגם מכלל דאינו קורא בתורה, וזה כונת ב"י בסי' קמ"א "דתנן סומא אין קורא בתורה דלא כאשכול". אבל האשכול ס"ל מדלא תנן בהדל' אין קורא בתורה כבשארא דמתני' דמשמע דאיכא אופן דקורא, שאם א' עומד בצדו וקורא מתוך הכתב יוכל הסומא לברך וקורא אחריו בע"פ.

49. Albeck explains the phantom Mishnah citation as follows:

גי הרי"ף במגילה פ"ד סי' אלף קמ"ב וה"ג ד"ב 225: סומא פורס על שמע וכו' "אבל אינו קורא בתורה", וכ"ה בתנחומא תולדות סי' ז עי"ש. ולפנינו במשנה כ"ד: הגי סומא פורס על שמע ומתרגם וכו' ותו לא, ובפוחח לפני זה הגי פורס את שמע ומתרגם אבל אינו קורא בתורה.

50. Albeck quotes *Beit Yosef,* and then conjectures the true intent of the Eshkol:

בב"י א"ח סי' קמא כתב: "דלא כדכתב נ"י בשם ספר האשכול דהא דתנן וכו' סומא אינו קורא בתורה היינו לומר דאינו קורא על פה, אבל אוקמו אינש אחרינא שפותח ורואה הסומא מברך ועומד בצדו ש"ד והכי מצי עביד חתן ומצאתי בשם ספר אגודה דסומא כהן קורא בתורה ואין לסמוך על דבריהם" וכו'. ולפי הלשון כאן אפשר שגם למחברנו אין הסומא מברך אלא האחר וצ"ע. ועי' בב"ח וט"ז שם ס"ק ג'.

51. I thank Rabbi Susan Grossman for this insight.

52. Susskind Goldberg, pp. 36-37.

53. Rabbi Alexander Zuslein HaKohen, d. Frankfurt, 1348.

54. ספר האגודה לבבא קמא, פרק החובל, סימן קד.

55. Rabbi David ben Samuel HaLevi, Ukraine and Poland, 1586-1667. Known by the title of his commentary, Taz, for *Turei Zahav*.

56. ט"ז מגן דוד. סימן קמא סעיף ג ס"ק ג.

57. The *Levush Malkhut (Royal Garment)* of Rabbi Mordechai b. Abraham Jaffee, Prague, Italy and Poland, c. 1535-1612.

58. Rabbi Joel Sirkes, known as the "BaCh" for the title of his commentary on the *Arba'ah Turim,* the *Bayit Chadash.* Poland, 1561-1640.

59. See also the Magen Avraham and Vilna Gaon to O.H. 49:1, and the sources cited there.

60. Germany, 1697-1776.

61. שאילת יעבץ חלק א סימן עה ד"ה ואמינא דהך.

62. שם בסוף הסימן. "ואילי גם מהרי"ל לא ס"ל הכי אלא מנהג הוא שהיו נוהגין כך בימיו, ולא הי' יכולת בידו למחות. כמו כמה מנהגים גרועים שיד ההמון תתקיף' על החכמים עשותה זאת ולא מעיקר הדין. אך ספר מהרי"ל אינו בידי כעת לדעת שורש דעתו."

63. שו"ת יביע אומר חלק ד-או"ח סימן ח ד"ה (טו) ובהיותי.

64. I thank Rabbi Roth for his detailed suggestions on this section.

65. ילקוט יוסף, ס' קלט, סדר הקריאה והברכות, ע' פד. ועיין בהערות.   I thank Rabbi Mayer Rabinowitz for this text.

66. ציץ אליעזר חלק יא (סימן י אות ב). "הרי לנו עדות נאמנה להתפשטות המנהג אצל קהילות הספרדים זי בכל אתר לקרוא סומא לס"ת גם לרבות בהרבה גלילות בחו"ל (על קהילות האשכנזים אין צורך להוכחה שקורים לסומא כי הרי יוצאים ביד רמ"א)."

67. שו"ת ציץ אליעזר שם. "ועל כן לפי דעתי לא טוב עשה בעמיו אותו ת"ח (שמזכיר בספרו) שביייש את הסומא הת"ח ומנע בעדו בריש גלי מלעלות לתורה, והוא רחום יכפר."

68. One sensitivity is to avoid calling the blind up for the second *aliyah* in *Emor* (Levit. 21:18) that discusses blindness as a disqualification for officiating priests, which could cause embarrassment to the *oleh.*

69. Rabbi Isaac Jacob Weiss (1902-1989). שו"ת מנחת יצחק חלק ג' סימן יב. However, Weiss agrees with Emden that the blind should not read Torah for the congregation nor even receive an *aliyah.*

70. A 1999 Master's thesis submitted to the H.L. Miller Cantorial School at the Jewish Theological Seminary by George Michael Horwitz contains a beautiful tribute to the careers of two blind cantors, Chazzan Moishele Soorkis (1900-1974) and Chazzan Todros Greenberg (1893-1976).

71. An Israeli company is developing a new computer mouse called VirTouch with similar touch pads that replicate in tactile contour the shape of objects on the screen. However, this would require use of a computer in the process of reading Torah.

72. הלכות תפילה פרק יב, הל' יז.

73. רמ"א שו"ע או"ח רפב, ס' ד.

74. See above, p. 13 and note 58.

75. In *Halachic Rulings for the Blind,* Rabbi David Toiv cites the Debreciner Rav, who "cautions that the ba'al koreh should read from the Torah at a slower pace, so that the blind can repeat the words after him."

76. מגילה כג ע"ב. ולהלכה ברמב"ם הלכות תפילה פרק י"ב הלכה י, ובטוש"ע א"ח ס' קמה סעיף א.

77. ב"ק ג ע"ב. ועיין בתוספות שם ד"ה כדמתרגם.

78. I thank Rabbi Joseph Prouser for this suggestion.

doi: 10.1300/J095v10n03_04

Reform Responsa Concerning Persons with Disabilities

Responsa Committee of the Central Conference of American Rabbis
with an Introduction by Rabbi Judith Z. Abrams, PhD

SUMMARY. The deciding body on individual questions of Jewish practice, the Responsa Committee of the Central Conference of American Rabbis, has issued many opinions on matters concerning disabilities over the years. This small, but representative, sample shows how the Reform Movement views responsibilities to those with disabilities and the rights of persons with disabilities to participate in Jewish life. doi:10.1300/J095v10n03_05 *[Article copies available for a fee from The Haworth Document Delivery Service: 1-800-HAWORTH. E-mail address: <docdelivery@haworthpress.com> Website: <http://www.HaworthPress.com>]*

KEYWORDS. Reform Judaism, disabilities, handicapped access, marital and parental responsibilities toward those with disabilities, blindness

INTRODUCTION

The tradition of asking questions of rabbinic authorities for guidance in dealing with specific problems is a venerated one in Jewish tradition. The liberal Reform Jewish movement has a Responsa Committee composed of rabbis belonging to the Central Conference of American Rabbis (the official organization of Reform Rabbis in North America). The

---

Rabbi Judith Z. Abrams is affiliated with Maqom: A School for Adult Talmud Study, Houston, TX.

[Haworth co-indexing entry note]: "Reform Responsa Concerning Persons with Disabilities." Responsa Committee of the Central Conference of American Rabbis, with an Introduction by Abrams, Rabbi Judith Z. Co-published simultaneously in *Journal of Religion, Disability & Health* (The Haworth Pastoral Press, an imprint of The Haworth Press, Inc.) Vol. 10, No. 3/4, 2006, pp. 53-72; and: *Jewish Perspectives on Theology and the Human Experience of Disability* (ed: Rabbi Judith Z. Abrams, and William C. Gaventa) The Haworth Pastoral Press, an imprint of The Haworth Press, Inc., 2006, pp. 53-72. Single or multiple copies of this article are available for a fee from The Haworth Document Delivery Service [1-800-HAWORTH, 9:00 a.m. - 5:00 p.m. (EST). E-mail address: docdelivery@haworthpress.com].

Available online at http://jrdh.haworthpress.com
doi:10.1300/J095v10n03_05

responsa below are a representative sample of the questions answered by the Responsa Committee concerning disabilities through the years. They are useful not only in addressing the individual question at hand but for marshalling textual sources that informed the committee's response. A comprehensive list of these responsa may be found at http://data.ccarnet.org/resp/tindex.html

CONTEMPORARY AMERICAN REFORM RESPONSA

202. Parental Obligation to a Severely Retarded Child

QUESTION: A couple with two healthy, normal children has a third child who is severely malformed and retarded. The child is not aware of people around him, and his intelligence is limited to a few reflexes. His face will occasionally form what appears to be a smile, and if food is placed in his mouth he will swallow by reflex. There is no hope for a future beyond this, however. The child has, for several years, simply lain in a fetal position in a crib in a nursing home. Do the parents have a continued obligation to visit this child or is it sufficient that they see to it that he is cared for in the institution where he now resides? Does the tradition provide some guidelines for determining the degree of medical care to be given to this child in a crisis? Physicians are generally surprised that the child has lived this long. If the reflex by which the child eats stops functioning, how far should the medical staff intervene to preserve life? Is there the obligation to feed him through a stomach tube, for example? (Rabbi M. Remson, Naperville, IL)

ANSWER: Let us begin by dealing individually with each question which you have asked. Traditional Judaism places an obligation for the maintenance of children upon the father; it is his duty to provide for all of his children's needs in accordance with his ability (*Yad* Ishut 13.6; *Shulhan Arukh* Even Haezer 73.6 ff). This includes formal education, learning a trade or anything else which will enable a child to take her place in the adult world (Kid. 29a ff; *Shulhan Arukh* Yoreh Deah 245.1, 4). There is some discussion about the number of years for which this obligation exists. Originally tradition limited it to six years (Ket. 49b, 65b; *Shulhan Arukh* Even Haezer 71.1) and indicated that after that time, the father was duty-bound to maintain the child as an act of *tzedaqah* (*Yad* Hil. Ishut 12.14, 15, 21.17; *Shulhan Arukh* Yoreh Deah 251.4). However, the demands of *tzedaqah* were to be enforced rigidly according to the actual needs of the child (*Yad* Hil. Ishut 13.6; *Shulhan Arukh* Even Haezer 73.6). This obligation then continues until age thirteen or in modern times until the child reaches an independent adult status.

Little has been said in our legal tradition about the emotional needs of the child, but such thoughts have been conveyed through the *aggadic* literature.

Nothing in the traditional literature limits such care to normal children. In other words, the obligation is universal and applies to every child regardless of her mental or physical abilities.

Tradition, therefore, indicates that this child, despite its very limited abilities, deserves both the maintenance and affection which the parents can provide. As I view this problem through my personal experience with a severely handicapped daughter and that of others who have dealt with parents of handicapped children, it is clear that unless ongoing relationships of some kind are established with such a handicapped child, the parents and other children will always feel guilty. Obviously this child can not be made part of the normal family life, but ongoing visits and continued concern with his welfare rests as any obligation upon all the members of the family. Practically speaking, such visits also assure a higher standard of care for such an individual, as those institutionalized children who receive no visits are frequently neglected.

Now, let me turn to the second portion of your question which asks about medical procedures in case this child's normal reflexes stop. We should follow the advice of the *Mishnah,* which states that no positive action which will hasten death may be instituted (*M.* Shab 23.5, 151b; *Shulhan Arukh* Yoreh Deah 339). On the other hand, the same sources indicate that we need not impede the individual's death when no recovery is possible. This matter has been discussed at some length by Solomon B. Freehof (W. Jacob, *American Reform Responsa,* # 77). Nothing unusual needs be done by the attending physician; there would be no obligation to feed this individual through a stomach tube, etc. We followed the decision with our own child.

In summary, as long as this handicapped child remains alive, he should be given all care and affection possible. If his reflexes stop and no recovery is possible, he should be permitted to die peacefully.

February 1984

NEW AMERICAN REFORM RESPONSA

43. Handicapped Access

QUESTION: My synagogue is interested in designing access to the building for the handicapped. We face unusual difficulties because of our landmarks status at Central Synagogue in New York. Although we have engaged an outstanding architect to prepare the plans and supervise the construction, some individuals connected with the historic landmark institutions object to any change in the building. What responsibilities does a synagogue have toward handicapped congregants? What does tradition say about this matter? (Rabbi Stanley M. Davids, New York NY)

ANSWER: The Jewish Biblical tradition, and later rabbinic tradition, dealt primarily with the deaf, the mute, and the blind (Lev. 19.14 ff). Rabbinic literature separated the deaf and mutes from the others as these individuals were considered unable to understand like the insane, and so incapable of participating in general or religious life (Hag 3.5; R H 29a; Eruv 31b; Hul 2a). For the lame no disabilities were indicated except that along with the blind they could not serve as priests (Lev 21.18); neither could anyone else with a permanent blemish. The blind were free from religious obligations (B K 87a; Kid 31a), but according to their ability were permitted to participate and lead services. So a blind *hazan* was permitted to officiate although he was not to read from the *Torah* (Meg 24a; Get 60b; *Yad* Hil Tef 8.12; *Shulhan Arukh* Orah Hayim 53.14; Git 60b). There was no discussion of other physical disabilities as such individuals have been considered part of the general community. They possessed all the rights and obligations of any other Jew including the obligation to pray with a *minyan* in a formal service (*Shulhan Arukh* Orah Hayim 90, 109, etc.; Peter S. Knobel (ed.) *Gates of Mitzvah* p. 12). No Jew could be excluded from religious service except in those rare occasions when the community used the *herem* as punishment (Rabenu Gershom Taqanot in Louis Finkelstein's *Jewish Self-Government in the Middle Ages,* pp. 120 f). Extraordinary steps have always been taken to assure a *minyan* for mourners and for those unable to attend synagogue services.

In the medieval period when synagogues were often located in a common courtyard, access could not be blocked in any way, nor could it be made difficult (Meir of Rothenburg *Responsa* #541, 542 *Shulhan Arukh* Orah Hayim 150).

Landmark status is important and serves us well in our effort to pre-serve historic synagogues and to maintain the Jewish artistic architec-tural tradition, however, the primary object of the synagogue is to serve all the members of our community. As the number of aged increases so will the number of individuals who are handicapped. It is an obligation for us to serve all segments of the community and to provide access to our synagogues for those who are handicapped.

December 1988

CCAR RESPONSA:
DIVORCE OF AN INCAPACITATED SPOUSE 5756.15

A couple in their thirties has been married for some years. The wife has contracted a debilitating and terminal disease, which by this point has left her bedridden and robbed her of the power of speech and com-munication. She is not comatose. She is aware of her surroundings, but she is unable to respond effectively to them. Her disease will inevitably lead to her death, but this is not imminent; the situation can continue for an extended period of time. The husband wishes to divorce his wife, on the grounds that she is no longer capable of fulfilling her role as a spouse. He stresses that he does not intend to abandon her; he will visit her on a regular basis, provide her with "emotional support," and pay her medical expenses. He insists, however, that his marriage is for all practical purposes at an end, and he wants to be free to marry again.

Does Jewish teaching support or oppose his desire for divorce? (Rabbi Richard A. Block, Los Altos Hills, CA)

Teshuvah

1. Reform Judaism and Divorce. Like all *she'elot* posed to us, this one requests that we provide an answer from the resources of "Jewish teaching." As such, some might think it strange that we, a committee of Reform rabbis, should entertain such an inquiry. It is well known, after all, that the Reform movement in North America recognizes civil di-vorce as a valid dissolution of marriage and does not require a *get* (or *get piturin*, a document of divorce at Jewish law) in order for either the wife or the husband to remarry.[1] It might therefore be argued that Reform Ju-daism defines divorce as a purely secular matter and would have little to say about the subject from a particularly religious perspective. In our view, this is a mistaken conclusion. Reform Judaism continues to regard divorce, as it regards marriage, a matter of *religious* concern and a legitimate object of "Jewish teaching."

The definition of divorce as a "secular" matter was adopted by the Philadelphia Conference of 1869, which resolved that "the dissolution of marriage is, on Mosaic and rabbinical grounds, a civil act only which never received religious consecration. It is to be recognized, therefore, as an act emanating altogether from the judicial authorities of the state. The so-called ritual *get* is in all cases declared null and void."[2] The theory was that as a civil act, divorce belongs to the traditional jurisprudential category of *dinei mamonot*, "monetary law," to which the rabbis have long applied the rule *dina demalkhuta dina*, "the law of the land is the law."[3] This view, put forth by R. Samuel Holdheim in Germany some two decades earlier,[4] was championed at the Conference by R. David Einhorn, who noted that "the Bible does not mention the bill of divorce (Deut. 24:1) as a subject of positive command, but only incidentally as a written instrument which the husband has to execute and deliver to the wife he intends to dismiss." Rabbinic Judaism, too, he continued, prescribes no benediction for the act of divorce as it does for marriage. Indeed:

When two persons unite in community for life, it is the function of religion to offer consecration, sanctification, and blessing . . . But if the holy bonds are severed, religion can only tolerate the act in sorrow and silence; it may offer consolation to the innocent sufferer or rebuke the conscience of the guilty, but certainly can not invest the act with its consecration.[5]

As an interpretation of Jewish law, the Holdheim-Einhorn theory is hardly free of difficulty. It is highly debatable that the *halakhah* considers divorce an aspect of monetary rather than of ritual law (*isur veheter*; *isura*).[6] The opposite is more likely the case, since divorce, like marriage, determines the personal status of the individuals involved and establishes such *ritual* prohibitions as forbidden marriage, adultery, incest, and illegitimacy. The 1869 resolution remains, nonetheless, the policy of the CCAR in theory as well as practice. With that, however, we stress that Reform Judaism has never been oblivious to the religious implications of divorce. For one thing, the Philadelphia Conference qualified its acceptance of civil divorce by stating that rabbis should refuse to remarry individuals divorced at civil law until they have studied the grounds upon which the divorces were granted: "Judaism recognizes the validity of divorce, then, only if the cause assigned is sufficient in conformity with the spirit of Jewish religion." One leading

Reform scholar went so far as to suggest that "a body of three rabbis should attest to the correctness from the Jewish point of view of the findings of the court in matters of divorce, and attach their signature to the bill of divorce issued by the court."[7] In other words, we as a religious body retain the power of supervision over divorce. While we have handed its administration over to the civil authorities, we have reserved to ourselves the right to judge whether their work is done "in a manner which is acceptable to us."[8] The Holdheim-Einhorn theory, moreover, may no longer strike us as persuasive on religious grounds. Today, we might argue that divorce, no less than marriage, warrants a religious response; that a union which originated in a religious ceremony demands some form of religious closure at the time of its dissolution; and that for Judaism to respond with mere "sorrow and silence" to such a fateful experience in the lives of couples and their children is an abdication of its religious responsibility. In recognition of these facts our movement has created a "Ritual of Release" which, though it does not take the place of the traditional *get*, serves as "a form of religious divorce" for couples who desire it[9] and "may eventually lead us to reopen the matter of a Reform *get*."[10]

Divorce, then, has never ceased to be a matter of *religious* concern to Reform Judaism. When we consider questions and problems relating to divorce, therefore, we do so not simply as counselors or pastors but as rabbis, scholars of Torah who draw their guidance from the sacred texts of our tradition. In the case before us, we shall need to consult the detailed halakhic discussions on the subject of grounds for divorce: would the husband in our *she'elah* be entitled, from the standpoint of Jewish law, to divorce his wife? We shall read these texts as Reform rabbis. This means that we seek to understand them in accordance with our commitment to gender equality and with the standards of justice and fairness to which we aspire in our personal and communal lives.

2. *Grounds for Divorce.* One way to think about this *she'elah* is to compare it to those cases in which our tradition recognizes the existence of valid grounds for divorce. Judaism holds divorce, like marriage, to be a private act, effected by the parties and not decreed by the court (*beit din*) or other legal agency. If both husband and wife agree to the divorce,[11] the role of the *beit din* is limited to supervising the details of the writing and delivery of the *get*. In cases where only one spouse seeks a divorce, however, the court is empowered to determine whether legitimate grounds exist to grant that request and to require the other spouse to acquiesce.

Our analysis assumes that the husband and his wife entered into no prior agreement authorizing divorce under circumstances such as these.[12] We shall inquire whether this situation is a valid grounds for divorce in the absence of explicit consent from either spouse.

The grounds for divorce in Jewish law can be classified into two categories: those based upon "objective" factors and those stemming from the inappropriate behavior of the other spouse. Among the "objective" factors are "defects" (*mumim*) in the spouse which render conjugal relations impossible.[13] Since the wife has a Toraitic right to conjugal relations,[14] certain blemishes, diseases, or occupations of her husband which cause her disgust and revulsion, to the point that she cannot bear to have sexual relations with him, can justify a finding for divorce.[15] In the case of the husband, traditional *halakhah* allows him to divorce his wife when she is afflicted with certain "defects" particular to women that preclude the possibility of conjugal relations.[16] Another "objective" factor is the husband's sexual impotence: if he cannot fulfill the *mitzvah* of conjugal relations, his wife is entitled to a divorce.[17]

Now to the present case. If we approach the question in this way, as an issue of "grounds for divorce," the husband would appear to have a strong claim. His wife, who as a result of her illness "is no longer capable of fulfilling her role as a spouse," cannot provide him with a functional "marital life" (*chayei ishut*). Jewish law regards the impossibility of conjugal relations, to which in our egalitarian reading of the tradition the husband and the wife are equally entitled,[18] as a legitimate warrant for the dissolution of a marriage. Based upon these considerations, we would be inclined to respond positively to the husband's argument.

3. Marriage, Disease, and Healing. There is, however, another way to understand this case from a traditional perspective. The *halakhah* declares that the husband is obligated under the terms of the marriage to provide his wife's medical expenses (*refu'ah*). Yet the *mishnah* which speaks of this requirement also offers a device whereby the husband can free himself of it: he is entitled to say "here is her *get* and her *ketubah*; let her heal herself."[19] He can, in other words, divorce his wife, thus limiting his liability for her medical treatment to the amount specified in the *ketubah* as the indemnity for divorce. This doctrine is extremely controversial in the law. While the leading codifiers adopt the *mishnah's* rule as authoritative, they add that "it is unethical" for the husband to divorce his wife under these circumstances.[20] Other authorities go farther, ruling on the basis of a passage in the *Sifre* that the husband does not enjoy this power at all and that he is not permitted to divorce his wife on account of her illness.[21] And in the opinion of R. Shelomo Luria

(Maharshal, an outstanding *posek* of 16th-century Poland), even if the husband has that power in theory he no longer enjoys it in practice. Today, under the edict of R. Gershom, a husband is prohibited from divorcing his wife without her consent. Therefore, under no circumstances may a husband use divorce to free himself of the requirement to provide her medical care.[22]

Seen in this light, our *she'elah* demands a negative response. The husband wishes to end his marriage due to his wife's illness. The sources, however, either condemn or explicitly prohibit divorce under such circumstances. The duty to provide for the healing of one's spouse[23] is part and parcel of the commitment of marriage and cannot be separated from the existence of the marital bond. It is therefore wrong to divorce one's spouse on account of the latter's illness.

4. Analysis. Our tradition, therefore, offers us two different approaches for thinking about our *she'elah*. Is the case before us one pertaining to "grounds for divorce"? Or should we perceive it as an instance of *refu'ah*, the duty to care for a spouse who is ill? We think that the latter of these two concepts affords the better understanding of the religious and moral aspects of the question.

In our view, the language of "defect" or "blemish" is inappropriate here. When the tradition speaks of *mumim* that are grounds for divorce, it refers to *particular* physical afflictions or *particular* occupations which are so loathsome or dangerous that the spouse is not expected to attempt to build a marital life with him or her. Such "defects" are understood as *exceptional* situations and are in no sense the norm in the population. Not every imaginable "defect" falls into this category;[24] those which do affect such a small proportion of the community that it can plausibly be argued that one is "entitled" to marry a spouse who is free of them. Disease, by contrast, including serious and even terminal disease, is an inescapable and universal element of the human condition. If a "defect" is an unusual and unacceptable departure from the norm or the average, disease *is* the norm for all creatures of flesh and blood. It is by no means an exceptional circumstance that one is "entitled" to avoid.[25]

The same can be said for "impotence," which we interpret as the physical or psychological inability of either spouse to engage in conjugal relations. The impotence which Jewish law recognizes as grounds for divorce was seen as a defect, the exception rather than the rule in human life.[26] The wife in this *she'elah* does not carry a "blemish." She is incapable of "fulfilling her role as a spouse" not because she suffers from the female equivalent of impotence but because she has become ill. Every single one of us becomes ill; we are all of us subject to diseases that may leave us unable to fulfill our marital and other responsibilities. And any one of us, prior to our death, may experience a protracted illness that renders us incapacitated for an extended period of time. These are unhappy realities, but they *are* realities, an inevitable part of the package called life. To say that we are somehow "entitled" to avoid these facts of human existence is tantamount to a claim that we are entitled to avoid marrying a spouse who will grow old and die. And that is patently absurd.

The question we should ask when confronting a situation such as this is not whether we enjoy the "right" to escape from it. We should rather inquire as to how our religious heritage and our most deeply-rooted moral values would have us respond to a spouse who lies on his or her deathbed. That responsibility, according to Jewish teaching, is not divorce but *refu'ah*, not abandonment but care and compassion. It is true that the husband in this instance promises to provide financial and emotional support to his wife following their divorce, and such good intentions are commendable. But we are not talking here about good intentions but about moral and ethical duty. Our tradition holds that it is marriage itself which creates this duty: *this* man is obligated to offer monetary and personal support to *this* woman precisely because they are united in a covenant of marriage which imposes responsibilities upon each spouse at the same time that it entitles them to "rights." Nowhere does Jewish law recognize "disease," even serious and incapacitating disease, as grounds for divorce. As befits a tradition which deplores divorce even though it allows it,[27] Judaism instead expects us to continue to fulfill the duties we accepted upon ourselves at the moment of *kidushin* and *nisu'in*.

This is a teaching we feel called upon to affirm. As liberals, participants in a culture that proclaims the rights and dignity of the individual person, we most certainly recognize the "right" to divorce. We understand that divorce can be an entirely proper alternative when a marriage has irrevocably broken down. But we also believe in marriage. We hold that the marital union remains a sacred commitment, a bond that ought to be broken only on valid "grounds," for the gravest of causes. And we cannot define the circumstances of this case as "grounds for divorce." On the contrary: precisely because the difficulty stems from the wife's illness, the correct response to it is *refu'ah*, a response which rules out divorce and which demands her husband's care, compassion, and continuing presence with her.

A final note. We are not unmindful of the anguish that this husband must be suffering. It is a painful thing to confront the decline and death of a loved one, and our *teshuvah* must not be read as an effort to minimize or belittle that pain. Our role in this question, however, is that of teachers of Torah, and the counsel we offer must reflect our best understanding of what Torah, the accumulated religious and moral experience of our people, would have us do when faced with this situation. And what Torah would have us do, we think, is to act in such a way that we leave no doubt as to our faithfulness to the values and to the commitments by which we measure the moral worth of our lives. To adhere to this standard may demand a high degree of personal sacrifice from us. Yet it is without question the best choice we can make.

Conclusion. Jewish tradition, as we understand and interpret it, does not recognize this husband's claim as sufficient grounds for divorce. Instead, it calls upon him to accept his responsibility to provide *refu'ah*, material and spiritual care, to his ailing wife.

NOTES

1. See *Ma`agalei Tzedek: Rabbi's Manual* (New York: CCAR, 1988), historical notes by W. Gunther Plaut, 244-246. We stress that this statement applies in general but not to every specific case. Suppose, for example, that a couple were married under the auspices of traditional Jewish law. In the event that their marriage ends in civil divorce, the husband's refusal to issue a *get* to his wife would render her an *agunah* and prevent her from remarrying according to *halakhah*. While we would recognize both parties as divorced and permitted to remarry, the husband's act is one of blatant injustice to his wife and a violation of his implicit promise, made at the time of *kidushin*, to accept the injunction of rabbinic law to execute a religious divorce when and if such is demanded. In such a circumstance, the husband should not be allowed to remarry in a Reform ceremony unless and until he executes the religious divorce. See our responsum 5754.6, *Teshuvot for the Nineties*, 209-215.

2. In R. Solomon B. Freehof, *Reform Jewish Practice I* (New York: UAHC Press, 1963), 107. Freehof, 99-110, provides a full discussion of the history of Reform thinking on the validity of civil divorce. See also R. Moses Mielziner, *The Jewish Law of Marriage and Divorce* (Cincinnati: Bloch, 1901), 130-137.

3. Freehof, 106. On the rule *dina demalkhuta dina* see our responsum 5757.1.

4. R. Samuel Holdheim, *Ueber die Autonomie der Rabbinen und das Princip der juedischen Ehe* (Schwerin/Berlin, 1843), 143*ff.*

5. Freehof, 106-107; Mielziner, 132-133.

6. See Mielziner, 131, citing R. Zechariah Frankel's critique of Holdheim's theory in *Zeitschrift fuer die religioesen Interessen des Judenthums*, 1:277*ff* (1844).

7. Freehof, 108. The leading Reform scholar was R. Kaufmann Kohler; see Freehof *loc. cit.* and *CCARY* 25 (1915), 377.

8. R. Walter Jacob, *Questions and Reform Jewish Answers*, no. 233, at 373.

9. For the "Ritual of Release" see *Rabbi's Manual*, 97-104. The citation "a form of religious divorce" appears at p. 245.

10. *QRJA*, no. 233, at 374.

11. The foregoing is a necessarily brief and incomplete description of the traditional Jewish law of divorce. In reality, while divorce is technically effected by both husband and wife, it is the husband who is the active party. It is he who writes or issues the *get* to the wife, whose role in the process is but to receive it. Thus, "the husband may divorce only with his consent; the wife can be divorced with or without her consent" (*BT* Gitin 49b; see Deut. 24:1 and *Yad*, Gerushin 1:2). The wife cannot divorce the husband. On the other hand, much of the history of the Jewish law of divorce has consisted of an effort to redress this imbalance. Rabbinic law permits the wife to "sue" for divorce on a variety of grounds and authorizes coercion of the husband, "with whips" if necessary, in order that he may "consent" to issue the *get* (*M.* Ketubot 7:10; *BT* Ketubot 77a-b; on the question of eliciting "consent" by means of force, see *Yad*, Gerushin 2:20). On all this, see further in the text. Moreover, the famous enactment (*cherem*) of Rabbenu Gershom b. Yehudah, "the Light of the Exile" (10th-11th cent., Mainz) forbids the husband from utilizing his Toraitic authority to divorce his wife without her consent (see Isserles, EHE 119:6). This enactment is accepted by Ashkenazim and by a number of other communities. It serves, writes one leading medieval authority, "to equate the power of the wife with that of the husband" in matters of divorce law (*Resp. R. Asher b. Yechiel* 42:1). While this estimate, sadly, is an exaggeration–the power to issue the *get* still rests exclusively with the husband, who can exploit that power to tragic effect–it does underline the tendency of the *halakhah* toward improving the legal status of the wife with respect to divorce. We Reform rabbis, committed to the principle of gender equality, simply propose to follow this tendency to the conclusion demanded by its inner logic and morality. Our analysis will assume as a matter of course that husband and wife shall function as equals throughout the divorce process.

12. Such an agreement would resemble the "conditional *get*" (*get al tena'i*), which takes effect only upon the meeting of certain specified stipulations; see *SA* EHE 143. Another possible analog is the "living will" in which individuals give their instructions to physicians and family members concerning their desires regarding medical treatment during the last stages of terminal illness. We mention these legal devices for purposes of comparison only; this is not the place for an extended discussion concerning either of them.

13. See Benzion Schereschewsky, *Dinei Mishpachah*, Third Edition (Jerusalem: Rubin Mass, 1984), 373*ff.*

14. Exodus 21:10; *BT* Ketubot 47b; *Yad*, Ishut 12:2.

15. The classic list of these *mumim* is preserved in *M.* Ketubot 7:10. In *BT* Ketubot 77a we read that the sign of some of these diseases is "a foul odor of the mouth or nose"; hence, the *halakhah* determines that the presence of "disgusting" symptoms ("so strong that one cannot bear them"; *Resp. R. Eliyahu Mizrachi* 2:19) justifies divorce. See *Yad*, Ishut 25:11-12 and *SA* EHE 154:1.

16. For example, a woman whose menstrual cycle is irregular to the point that she is never certain as to when she is a *nidah* (*BT* Nidah 12b; *Yad*, Ishut 25:7-9).

17. *BT* Yevamot 65a. The details of this issue are spelled out in *SA* EHE 154:6-7.

18. The sources do not speak of an "obligation" on the part of the wife to provide sexual relations to the husband, but rather of *his* obligation to do so for her. For us, this gender-based distinction carries no relevance. We would regard both parties to the marriage as equally entitled and equally obligated in the realm of *chayei ishut.*

19. *M.* Ketubot 4:9. See Bartenura *ad loc.*: he is entitled to do this because "a man is not obligated to provide maintenance (*mezonot*) to his divorcee," and the duty of *refu'ah* is considered a subset of *mezonot.* See *BT* Ketubot 52b.

20. *Yad,* Ishut 14:7; *SA* EHE 79:3. See *Magid Mishneh* to *Yad ad loc.*: it is "obvious" that for the husband to use this power is an affront to ethical standards.

21. This view is found in the *chidushim* of Rashba and Ritva to *BT* Ketubot 52b and is attributed to R. Avraham b. David of Posquierres (Rabad). See also Meiri *ad loc.* The *Sifre* passage is ch. 214 (to Deut. 21:14), which states that the Israelite soldier may not send away his female captive of war (*eshet yefat to'ar*) while she is ill. The *midrash* reasons that if this is the case with the captive, whom the Torah with great reluctance permits one to marry (see *BT* Kidushin 21b and Rashi to Deut. 21:11), then it is certainly true of one's wife. Rabad, noting the contradiction between this passage and *M.* Ketubot 4:9, suggests that the *mishnah*'s rule applies only when the wife is not seriously ill.

22. Maharshal's ruling is cited in *Bayit Chadash* to *Tur,* EHE 79, fol. 102a, and in *Beit Shmuel* to *SA* EHE 79, no. 4. On the edict (*cherem*) of R. Gershom, see note 11, above.

23. Again, we stress our egalitarian reading of the tradition. In our view the duty of *refu'ah* is as incumbent upon the wife as it is upon the husband.

24. For example, should a husband become blind or lose a limb his wife is not entitled by that reason to a divorce, even though such conditions are described as "serious defects" (*mumim gedolim*). See *M.* Ketubot 7:9; *BT* Ketubot 77a; *Yad,* Ishut 25:11; *SA* EHE 154:4.

25. Indeed, we are not always entitled to avoid even those *mumim* that are accepted as grounds for divorce. For example, if a wife knew about the "defect" prior to marriage or continued to live with her husband following its discovery, some authorities rule that "she thought about it and accepted it" (*savrah vekiblah*), thus waiving her right to divorce (*BT* Ketubot 76a; *Yad,* Ishut 25:11; Isserles, EHE 154:1). With respect to *mumim* in the wife, the tradition holds that should these "defects" develop subsequent to marriage the husband has no claim to divorce. The principle is *nistachfah sadehu* (literally, "his field has flooded," an occurrence which Western legal tradition would call "an act of God"): it is the husband's fate that this has happened, and there is nothing he can do to remedy the situation. See *BT* Ketubot 75a; *Yad,* Ishut 25:9-10; *SA* EHE 117:1.

26. The use of the past tense in this sentence is indicative of today's awareness that "impotence" is a condition that can be treated with medical or psychological therapies. "Impotence," in this regard, may not be an automatic grounds for divorce; see *SA* EHE 76, the glosses of *Chelkat Mechokek,* no. 18, and *Beit Shmuel,* no. 17.

27. See *M.* Gitin 9:10. The talmudic discussion (*BT* Gitin 90a-b) leads to the conclusion that "a man should not divorce his first wife unless she has acted as a harlot" (*Yad,* Gerushin 10:21; *SA* EHE 119:3). Moreover, "when a man divorces his first wife, even the altar sheds tears on his account" (*BT* Gitin 90b).

CCAR RESPONSA 5759.8

A Blind Person as a Witness

She'elah

From a traditional and from a Reform perspective, may a blind person serve as a witness at a wedding? (Rabbi Joseph Forman, Elkins Park, PA)

Teshuvah

We say "yes" to this question, though traditional *halakhah* would likely answer it in the negative. Maimonides includes the blind among the ten persons disqualified from serving as witnesses before a court.[1] The exclusion, he tells us, is Toraitic, derived by way of a midrash on Leviticus 5:1. The verse speaks of a public adjuration (*kol alah*) imposing a requirement to testify upon "one who has either seen or learned of the matter." Since blind persons have not "seen" the matter, they are exempted from the responsibility of giving testimony upon it.[2] The ceremony of betrothal (*kidushin*), if it is to be valid according to Jewish law, must occur in the presence of two witnesses[3] who see the transfer of the ring from groom to bride.[4] These witnesses must meet the standards of eligibility demanded of all witnesses; should either or both of them be among the ten "disqualified witnesses" (*pesulei edut*) mentioned above, it is as though no testimony exists and the wedding is invalid.[5]

Our contrary viewpoint is based upon the following three arguments. First, it is quite possible that the *halakhah* recognizes the validity of a marriage even when the wedding ceremony is conducted in the presence of ineligible witnesses. Second, despite the description of the law in the preceding paragraph, a case can yet be made that blind persons are *not* to be disqualified from serving as witnesses to a wedding. And third, as Reform Jews, we endorse the general tendency of Jewish law to include the blind in religious life to the greatest extent possible.

1. Valid Testimony Without Qualified Witnesses. Our first point is the subject of a responsum by R. Moshe Sofer ("Chatam Sofer," d. 1839).[6] The case concerns a wedding at which the officiating rabbi (the *mesader kidushin*) designated himself and the local synagogue sextant (*shamash*) as the witnesses to the ceremony. Some weeks later, the rabbi discovered that the *shamash* was a relative of the bride and hence disqualified to serve as a witness concerning her.[7] Should he require that a second wedding ceremony be held in the presence of two qualified witnesses, or is it sufficient that the first ceremony was conducted in the presence of a large assembly of people (including a number of rabbis) who, though they did not witness the actual exchange of the ring (the *ma'aseh kidushin*), could at least testify that a wedding ceremony did take place? Sofer responded that the wedding ceremony was valid on the basis of the concept *anan sahadei* ("we are all witnesses").[8] Since the couple entered the *chupah* in the presence of numerous qualified witnesses–among whom were the rabbi and other individuals knowledgeable of the law–with the obvious intention to marry, and since the couple left the *chupah* under the unchallenged presumption (*chazakah*) that they were married, "then surely 'we are all witnesses' to the fact that a valid act of *kidushin* took place, including the transfer of the ring and the proper verbal formula, following the instructions of the officiating rabbi who is knowledgeable of the laws concerning marriage." The fact that one of the designated witnesses under the *chupah* turned out to be ineligible does not invalidate this testimony, based upon the common knowledge of the wider community.[9] Similarly, R. Yosef Eliyahu Henkin, one of the outstanding twentieth-century *poskim* in the United States, ruled that if no witnesses are present at the wedding, the marriage of two Jews is still valid according to *halakhah* by virtue of the fact that they live together in public as husband and wife. Thus, "common knowledge" is sufficient testimony that a wedding has taken place and that a marriage exists.[10]

"Common knowledge" also suffices to establish a valid marriage in cases where the witnesses do not actually see a vital aspect of the transaction. For example, it is a custom in some circles for the bride's face to be veiled during the wedding ceremony. The question is raised: since the witnesses in such a case do not actually see her face, how can they identify her as the bride, the one who accepted the *kidushin* from the groom? Is a second act of *kidushin* required to validate the marriage? Some say "yes," that the marriage cannot be declared valid when the witnesses did not actually see the bride's face.[11] Most authorities, however, side with the author of the commentary *Avnei Milu'im*,[12] who holds that such testimony is valid.[13] He writes: "we require the testimony of witnesses to a wedding only in order to make the fact of the marriage public knowledge, so that neither party can deny the wedding took place." Since the identity of the wife will become public knowledge as soon as the wedding is ended, it is as though the witnesses had seen her at the actual moment of *kidushin*. The presumption (*chazakah*) that the wife was in fact the one standing under the *chupah* substitutes for actual eyewitness testimony.[14]

Thus, while testimony (*edut*) is an absolute requirement for determining the legal validity of a wedding, this testimony may be established by "common knowledge" as well as by the presence at the wedding of two "kosher" witnesses. The authors of these rulings do not, of course, mean to say that it is perfectly permissible to invite disqualified witnesses to perform that function at a wedding. These cases involve situations that are *bedi`avad*, "after the fact." In principle (*lekhatchilah*), these authorities would demand that the officiating rabbi make sure in advance of the wedding that the witnesses are qualified under *halakhah* to give testimony. Yet so long as it is "common knowledge" that the couple have married, we need not demand the testimony of two qualified witnesses in order to declare their marriage valid.

2. *The Blind as Qualified Witnesses*. Although, as we have seen, Maimonides rules that the blind are disqualified as witnesses on the basis of Torah law, the Talmud offers an alternative theory as to their disqualification. We find this in *BT* Gitin 23a, which discusses the *mishnah's* ruling that a blind person is not permitted to act as the agent for transporting a bill of divorce (*get*) from the husband to the wife.[15] The Talmud inquires as to the reason for this disqualification. Rav Sheshet responds: "because a blind person cannot tell from whom he receives the *get* and to whom he gives it." His colleague, Rav Yosef, rejects this argument: "if so, then why is a blind man permitted to live with his wife? Surely this is because he recognizes her voice; in the case of a *get* as well, a blind person might be able to identify the sender and receiver by their voices (and thus be eligible to transport the document)." Rather, concludes Rav Yosef, this *mishnah* deals with a *get* sent to the land of Israel from the Diaspora; in such a case the agent must be able to testify that "this document was written and signed in my presence."[16] That is, the blind person is disqualified simply because this particular agency requires that the agent actually see the persons who commission the *get*. The implication is that a blind person might well be accepted as a witness to matters upon which he can speak reliably and that do not require eyewitness knowledge. This conclusion, writes R. Barukh Halevy Epstein (d. 1942), runs directly counter to that of Maimonides. According to the latter, the Torah disqualifies the blind from serving as witnesses simply because they cannot see; a blind person may therefore never testify, even to matters that do not require eyesight. By contrast, should we follow the approach taken in Gitin 23a, we might conclude

that "there is a logical basis (*sevara*) to say that a blind person may testify" on matters that can be established by means other than eyesight.[17]

We agree with this logic. Since it is not absolutely certain that Maimonides is correct–that the Torah disqualifies the blind from testifying on *all* matters–there does not seem to be any good reason to deny them the right and the duty to serve as witnesses in matters that do not require eyewitness testimony. A wedding partakes of this latter category. Although a blind person cannot see the wedding transaction, so long as he or she recognizes the couple by their voices, can follow the exchange of rings by touching their hands during the moment of *kidushin*, and can hear them recite the formulae of marriage (*harei at/ah mekudeshet/mekudash, etc.*), he or she can reliably testify that a wedding has indeed taken place.

3. Inclusion of the Blind in Jewish Religious Life. We should remember as well that Jewish law does not as a general rule seek to exclude or exempt the blind from the circumference of religious obligation. Despite the view of an early rabbinical authority to the contrary,[18] the accepted *halakhah* requires the obligated to fulfill the *mitzvot*, exempting them only from those duties and experiences that require eyesight.[19] Concerning those exemptions, moreover, the tradition has demonstrated that it is capable of change, bringing the blind into the orbit of an observance from which they were originally excluded. The question whether a blind person may be "called up" (given an *aliyah*) to the public reading of the Torah is a case in point. Originally, those who were called up to the Torah were the ones who actually performed the reading.[20] Since the text must be read directly from the scroll and not from memory, the person called to the Torah (the *oleh*) must possess the ability to read it, even if he assigns that task to a designated reader (*chazan* or *ba'al keri'ah*).[21] For this reason, a number of leading authorities prohibit a blind person from being called to the Torah.[22] Yet others dissent from this ruling on the grounds that, since the *ba'al keri'ah* is in fact the one who performs the reading, we do not insist that the *oleh* be capable of reading on his own. It is enough that he (and now she) recite the benedictions and stand by the *ba'al keri'ah*.[23] The blind may therefore be "called up" to the Torah, and such has long been the accepted practice.[24]

The example of the public reading offers a particularly helpful analogy to our case. At a time in history when the Torah was read by those "called up" to the scroll, those who could not physically read from the scroll were quite appropriately excluded from this observance. Over the years, the nature of this ritual changed: those "called up" to the scroll were no longer expected to perform the reading themselves. Accordingly, the exclusion no longer made sense, and the blind were allowed to participate. In a similar way, our understanding of the nature of "wedding testimony" (*edut kidushin*) has also changed. Given that the *halakhah* is prepared to accept "common knowledge" as sufficient testimony that a wedding has taken place, and given that "there is a logical basis" upon which to conclude that the blind may offer testimony on matters that do not–strictly speaking–require eyesight, a good argument can be made that it no longer makes sense to exclude blind persons from this aspect of Jewish ritual life.

As Reform Jews, we regard it a positive duty to include the blind and all others who are physically disabled in the activities of our congregations and communities. We base this affirmation, in part, upon the traditional insight that to exclude the blind from the *mitzvot* is to exclude them from Jewish experience altogether.[25] Our movement's historic commitment to the cause of social justice transforms this insight into a call to action: it is our obligation to do whatever we can to remove barriers that prevent the disabled from participating as fully as possible in Jewish life.[26] In this case, since Jewish text and tradition *can* be understood so as to permit the blind to serve as witnesses to a wedding, we must adopt that understanding as our own. So long as a blind person, through the use of the senses of hearing and touch, can identify the bride and the groom and can testify that the act of *kidushin* has taken place, we must permit them the opportunity to do so.

NOTES

1. *Yad*, Edut 9:1. The full list: women, slaves, children, the insane, the deaf-mute, the blind, the wicked, the despised (*bezuyin*, "uncouth" or "shameless"; see *Yad*, Edut 11:5), relatives, and those who are implicated in their own testimony.

2. *Yad*, Edut 9:12. The midrash is found in *Tosefta* Shevu`ot 3:6.

3. *BT* Kidushin 65b; *Yad,* Ishut 4:6; *SA* EHE 42:2.

4. Isserles, EHE 42:2.

5. *Yad*, Ishut 4:6; *SA* EHE 42:5. The validity of the wedding depends upon the nature of the witness's disqualification. If the witness is disqualified by Torah law (*mide'oraita*), the wedding is certainly invalid; if the disqualification is based upon rabbinic ordinance (*miderabanan*), the *halakhah* may require a divorce before permitting the parties to remarry. See *Magid Mishneh* to *Yad ad loc.*

6. *Resp. Chatam Sofer*, EHE 100.

7. The disqualification of witnesses is derived from the verse Deut. 24:16. See *M.* Sanhedrin 3:1 and 4; *BT* Sanhedrin 27b; and *Yad* Edut 13:1.

8. See *BT* Bava Metzi`a 3a and 4a. This principle is invoked in cases where the court will rely upon estimate (*umdana*), legal presumption (*chazakah*), or custom

(*minhag*) to establish facts, so that no direct or eyewitness testimony (*edut berurah*) is required.

9. Sofer deduces his conclusion from the commentary of R. Nissim Gerondi to the *Halakhot* of Alfasi, Gitin, fol. 47b-48a. There are two types of witnesses to the procedure of divorce: the *eidei mesirah*, those who witness the transmission of the *get* from husband to wife, and the *eidei chatimah*, the witnesses to the writing of the *get* who sign their name thereto. The *halakhah* follows Rabbi Eleazar, who holds that the *get* becomes valid because of the *eidei mesirah* and that the witnesses to the writing of the *get* are necessary only as a precaution, in the event that the *eidei mesirah* should be unavailable to testify that the *get* was properly handed to the wife (*M.* Gitin 4:3 and 9:4; *BT* Gitin 36a; *Yad,* Gerushin 1:15). R. Nissim suggests, however, that even Rabbi Eleazar would accept the validity of the *get* based upon the signatures alone. This is not because those signatures themselves validate the *get*; only the witnesses to its transmission accomplish that. Rather, the signatures allow us to conclude that this *get* was properly filled out before a qualified *beit din*, so that (in Sofer's words) "we all know that the document passed from the husband to the wife. Even if witnesses did not see this transmission, we are all witnesses to the transmission." In other words, though there is no actual testimony to the act of transmission—and it is upon that act that the *get*'s validity depends—our common knowledge allows us to presume with confidence that a proper transmission took place. Sofer applies this logic to the case of witnesses to the wedding.

10. Henkin makes this point in the following works: *Teshuvot Ibra*, no. 76; *Lev Ibra*, pp. 14-15; and *Perushei Ibra*, ch. 2.

11. See especially R. Moshe Trani (16th century), *Resp. Mabit* 1:226: since at the time of the wedding there was no firm knowledge of the identity of the one who accepted the *kidushin*, the discovery of her identity at a later point does not retroactively validate the marriage. We require knowledge at the time of the wedding itself.

12. *Avnei Milu'im* 31, no. 4.

13. See *Otzar Haposkim*, EHE 42:4, no. 22, for an exhaustive list of these authorities.

14. And see R. Eliezer Waldenberg, *Resp. Tzitz Eliezer* 11:82, at p. 216.

15. *M.* Gitin 2:5. The technical term for such as agent is *shaliach leholakhah*.

16. *M.* Gitin 1:1.

17. *Torah Temimah* to Lev. 5:1, no. 18.

18. *BT* Bava Kama 87a.

19. Thus, the blind are included in the practice of *tzitzit*, even though they cannot see the fringes on the four corners of their garments (*SA* OC 17:1); the blind may lead the *tefilah* (*SA* OC 53:14) as well as the *Shema* for the congregation (*SA* OC 69:12). On the other hand, the blind do not recite the blessing "who has created the lights of the fire" at *havdalah*, since one must be able to make use of the light before reciting this benediction (*SA* OC 298:13; yet they are permitted to recite the other benedictions of the *havdalah* service; see *Mishnah Berurah ad loc.*). A blind person may not serve as a *shochet* under ordinary circumstances (*SA* Yore De`ah 1:9). Finally, a blind person is not permitted to read from the Torah as part of a public service (*SA* OC 53:14), since one must be able to read the words of Torah from the actual text. On this, however, see below.

20. On the history of this practice, see Ismar Elbogen, *Jewish Liturgy: A Comprehensive History* (Philadelphia-New York: Jewish Publication Society/Jewish Theological Seminary, 1993), 140-141.

21. "Words of Torah that are written down may not be recited from memory"; *BT* Gitin 60b. Thus, "it is forbidden to read aloud from the Torah even one word not directly from the text;" *Yad*, Tefilah 12:8.

22. *SA* Orach Chayim 53:14 and 139:3; *Tur* and *Beit Yosef*, Orach Chayim 141. Similarly, an illiterate person should not be called to the Torah, since he cannot read from the text. He is not permitted, therefore, to recite a blessing over the *chazan*'s recitation of the Torah unless he himself can discern the letters and read them along with the *chazan*. See R. Asher b. Yechiel, *Resp. Harosh* 3:12, and R. Yitzchak b. Sheshet Perfet, *Resp. Rivash*, no. 204.

23. R. Ya`akov Molin (15th-century Germany), *Sefer Maharil*, Hil. Keri'at Hatorah, no. 3; Isserles, *SA* OC 139:3; R. Binyamin Selonik (16th-century Poland), *Resp. Masat Binyamin*, no. 62; R. Mordekhai Yaffe (16th-century Poland), *Levush*, OC 141:3; *Magen Avraham*, OC 139, no. 4; *Turey Zahav*, OC 141, no. 3.

24. *Mishnah Berurah*, OC 139, no. 13; *Arukh Hashulchan*, OC 139, par. 3.

25. See Tosafot, *Bava Kama* 87a, *s.v. vekhen haya R. Yehudah potero mikol hamitzvot*: "if you exempt the blind from the requirement to observe all the commandments, even if this requirement is rabbinically-imposed, you make him as though he is a Gentile, who does not walk in the path of Judaism at all."

26. This Committee has written that the inclusion of the disabled in our synagogues and other Jewish institutions is itself a *mitzvah*, an obligation that demands concrete action on our part. See *Teshuvot for the Nineties*, no. 5752.5.

doi: 10.1300/J095v10n03_05

SCHOLARLY APPROACHES

Misconceptions About Disabilities
in the Hebrew Bible

Rabbi Judith Z. Abrams, PhD

SUMMARY. The passages in the Torah referring to the physical perfection required of priests (Leviticus 21:16-24) are often erroneously understood to refer to all Israelites. Not only are these standards required
only of priests, once the Temple was destroyed these standards were gradually relaxed in connection with the most salient priestly activity left: the
priestly benediction. doi:10.1300/J095v10n03_06 *[Article copies available for a fee
from The Haworth Document Delivery Service: 1-800-HAWORTH. E-mail address:
<docdelivery@haworthpress.com> Website: <http://www.HaworthPress.com>
© 2006 by The Haworth Press, Inc. All rights reserved.]*

Rabbi Judith Z. Abrams is affiliated with Maqom: A School for Adult Talmud
Study, Houston, TX (E-mail: maqom@compassnet.com).

[Haworth co-indexing entry note]: "Misconceptions About Disabilities in the Hebrew Bible." Abrams,
Rabbi Judith Z. Co-published simultaneously in *Journal of Religion, Disability & Health* (The Haworth Pastoral Press, an imprint of The Haworth Press, Inc.) Vol. 10, No. 3/4, 2006, pp. 73-84; and: *Jewish Perspectives
on Theology and the Human Experience of Disability* (ed: Rabbi Judith Z. Abrams, and William C. Gaventa)
The Haworth Pastoral Press, an imprint of The Haworth Press, Inc., 2006, pp. 73-84. Single or multiple copies
of this article are available for a fee from The Haworth Document Delivery Service [1-800-HAWORTH, 9:00
a.m. - 5:00 p.m. (EST). E-mail address: docdelivery@haworthpress.com].

KEYWORDS. Disabilities, priests, priestly benediction, physical perfection

When one gazes at something a far way off, one's perspective is altered and the true distance can be foreshortened. This is a problem not only with physically seeing something but also when trying to understand something that is far removed from us in time. Scholars often casually explain whole centuries with a few broad strokes while, in contrast, historical events between 1941-1945 showed such dynamic changes that whole libraries are filled with descriptions of these years. It is logical to assume that society continually underwent such transmogrifications that were likely to have been part of ancient life as well. Biblical texts are, obviously, included in this category. Indeed, particularly when it comes to issues such as the physical perfection of priests or the role of disabilities in the Bible, we must overcome the distance of 3,000 years or more. It is the purpose of this paper to clarify the intention of the Biblical and rabbinic authorships regarding some teachings about disabilities that are often terribly misunderstood today.

ABILITIES AND DISABILITIES COME FROM GOD

One of the most salient passages for understanding the Torah's theology of disabilities arises when Moses protests to God that he cannot lead the Israelites from slavery to freedom because he has a speech impediment.

> And Moses said unto the Lord: My Lord, I am not a man of words, neither yesterday nor the day before nor ever since you have spoken to your servant, for I am slow of speech and slow of tongue. And God said to him, "Who puts a mouth in a person? And who makes him mute or deaf or seeing or blind? Is it not I, the Lord? (Exodus 4:10-11)

The meaning is clear: God is the provider of all human faculties. God is perceived as responsible not only for the proper functioning of the body, but also for those aspects which mark it as living:

> Our Rabbis taught: There are three partners in a person, the Holy One, blessed be He, his father and his mother. His father sows the

white [substance, i.e., semen] out of which [come the child's] bones and sinews and nails and the brain in his head and the white in his eye; his mother sows the red [substance, i.e. blood] out of which [come the child's] skin and flesh and hair and blood and the black of the eye. And the Holy One, blessed be He, gives him spirit and breath and beauty of face and seeing eyes and hearing ears and walking legs and understanding and insight. When the time comes for him to depart from the world, the Holy One, blessed be He, takes away His portion and leaves the portions of his father and mother with them. (B. Niddah 31a//B. Kiddushin 30b)

The contributions of man and woman reflect the "output" with which they are associated: white/semen from men and red/blood from women. God is an integral partner with man and woman in the genesis of a human body. What God contributes are the faculties: the ability to see, hear, speak, walk and understand, in other words, what makes a human being unique among God's creatures.

THE PRIESTS' PERFECTION IN THE TEMPLE

The most common misconception about disabilities in the Bible is that the rules for physical perfection which apply to priests also apply to all other Israelites. Such a notion is utterly incorrect. Complete priestly physical perfection applied only to priests officiating in the Temple.

To understand the role of a priest in the Temple–and the need for a priest to be blemishless in his physical form and lineage–we must understand the symmetry between heaven and earth and how crucial the priest was in mediating between the upper and lower realms. The world is full of death, disorder and imperfection. In heaven there is eternal life, order and perfection. Only in the Temple could these two realms come into contact. The priest, then, had to stand in two worlds at once. He had to be worthy of the heavenly beings whose company he shared and had to be able to survive coming into direct contact with God which was ordinarily considered lethal.

Access to the Sanctuary of the Temple was severely limited precisely because of the danger which was liable to befall those who approached this holy area improperly. Even if one's motives and intentions were of the most pious sort, the danger was still present. Holiness is "blindly" lethal in this sense. This may best be seen in the story of Nadav and Avihu.

> And the sons of Aaron, Nadav and Avihu, each took his fire pan and they put fire in them and placed upon them incense and offered before God a strange fire which they had not been commanded to offer. And fire came out from before God and consumed them and they died before God. (Leviticus 10:1-2)

No motive is imputed for Nadav and Avihu's offering of incense which God did not command. Yet the conclusion is clear: whether one's motives are good or bad is irrelevant in the lethal atmosphere of the Holy of Holies.

One relatively late source confirms the lethal nature of God's presence which resides in a synagogue made of stones from the first Temple's ruins. It involves one of the most prominent sages of Babylonia, Rav Sheshet (290-320 C.E.) who was blind. In this case, his disability actually protects him from God's lethal presence, from which other sages must flee.

> Rav Sheshet was [once] sitting in the synagogue which "moved and settled" in Nehardea, when God's presence approached. He did not go out [of the synagogue as did other sages]. The ministering angels came and [tried to] scare him [away]. He [Rav Sheshet] said to Him [God]: "Master of the Universe, if one is afflicted and one is not afflicted, who gives way to whom?" God [then] said to them [the angels]: "Leave him." (B. Megillah 29a)

The assumption behind this story is clear: God's presence is awful in every sense of that word and human beings must flee from it. Rav Sheshet, not being able to flee, asked for, and was granted, mercy. Perhaps the greatest part of God's holiness was conveyed through sight (sight > blinding insight). Rav Sheshet clearly has great insight and is enlightened, though physically blind.

To survive in such a dangerous position, the priest had to be fit for the company of God and angels, i.e., blemishless, pure of lineage and untouched by the taint of death or dysfunction (i.e., ritually pure).

> And the Lord spoke to Moses, saying: Speak to Aaron, saying, a man of your lineage, for [all] their generations, who has a blemish, shall not come near to offer the bread of his God. For any man who has a blemish shall not come near: [whether he] is a blind man or a lame man or [has] a flat nose or any extra [limb or growth] or a man who has a broken leg or a broken hand or a crooked back or

[is] a dwarf or has obscured sight in [even one] eye or has scurvy or scabs or crushed testicles. Any man of Aaron's lineage who has a blemish shall not draw nigh to offer the fire [offerings] of God. He has a blemish and the bread of his God come near to offer the offerings of the Lord made by fire: he has a blemish and he should not draw nigh to offer the bread of his God. He shall eat the bread of his God, [both] of the most holy, and of the holy. But he may not go [in] to the veil [before the ark], nor come near to the altar, because he has a blemish. Let him not profane My holy [places]: for I the Lord [Myself] sanctify [these places]. And Moses spoke [these words] to Aaron and to his sons and to all the children of Israel. (Leviticus 21:16-24)

The list of blemishes which disqualify sacrificial animals is, like those for the priest, twelve in number:

And a man who offers a peace offering to God, to fulfill a vow or whosoever brings a sacrifice of peace-offerings unto the Lord in fulfillment of a vow or for a free-will offering, of the herd or of the flock, it [must] be perfect to be accepted; it may have no blemish. Blind or broken[-limbed], or maimed or having a wen or scabbed or scurvy; do not sacrifice [such as] these to God nor make a fire [offering] to God of them on the altar for God. Either a bullock or a lamb that has any thing too long or too short, that may offer for a freewill-offering; but for a vow it shall not be accepted. That which has its testicles bruised, or crushed, or torn or cut you must not offer to God, nor may you perform [castrations] in your land. (Leviticus 22:21-24)

Five items in these lists are identical: blind, overgrown limb, broken bones, sores and scabs. Animals that were not fit to be sacrifices could still be eaten just as Israelites with disabilities could still come to the Temple bringing their sacrifices.

Priests with disabilities could still maintain their status even though they were unable to function in the Temple. Leviticus 22:1-16 outlines those special offerings that only a priest and his family could eat (*terumah*). These offerings could only be consumed by members of priestly families who were in a state of ritual purity. A priest who had a blemish which barred him from officiating in the cult could still eat these offerings (Leviticus 21:22). These rules redefined disability in terms of what that would mean to a priest. If a priest had a defective lineage he would be utterly disqualified from officiating at the cult and from receiving *terumah*. A state of ritual impurity would likewise deprive him of these same benefits although only for as long as the state of impurity lasted.

To reiterate: the main misconception that should be laid to rest here is that the physical perfection demanded of priests had nothing to do with the rest of the population. Persons with disabilities were as welcome as anyone to bring sacrifices to the Temple compound and to participate in the service. A close reading of these texts shows how few individuals were affected by these requirements of physical perfection.

Indeed, after the Temple's destruction, the sages showed how even one without special lineage (or even damaged lineage) could be greater than a priest:

> A priest takes precedence over a Levite; a Levite over an Israelite; an Israelite over a bastard . . . This order of precedence applies only when they were equal in all other respects. If the bastard, however, is a scholar and the High Priest an ignoramus, the learned bastard takes precedence over the ignorant High Priest. (M. Horayot 13a)

THE PRIESTS' PERFECTION
AFTER THE TEMPLE'S DESTRUCTION

When the Temple was destroyed in 70 C.E., the main locus of the priests' functioning was gone. They could, however, continue to function as priests in a few limited circumstances. One of these venues was when they uttered the priestly benediction during worship services in the synagogue. To this day, priests from the congregation come forward, shed their shoes, have their hands washed with the help of those who have descended from the Levites and ascend the *bimah* (platform) to bless the congregation with the words of Numbers 6:24-26. As part of this ritual, the priests raise their hands over the congregation. God's presence is believed to descend upon the priests' hands while this blessing is being offered. Hence, congregants are not supposed to look at the priests while the blessing is being recited lest this prove fatal. We see, then, that in this ritual moment, the atmosphere of lethal holiness that always obtained in the Temple is recreated in the synagogue.

The priests recited this benediction as part of the Temple service. Is it logical, then, to assume that when this ritual was performed in the synagogue that the priest must be blemishless? The requirement of physical perfection was applied to only a limited extent, i.e., their hands should be free of defects:

> A priest whose hands have blemishes may not raise his hands [in the priestly blessing]. Rabbi Yehudah says, "Moreover one whose hands are stained with woad [blue dye] or madder [red dye] may not lift his hands because the people would gaze at him. (M. Megillah 4:7)

When the priest lifts his hands in blessing the congregation, the Mishnah (200 C.E.) holds that the priest's hands must be blemishless. Not only that, even perfectly formed hands are not sufficient: they must also have the correct color. The concern here is that the congregation would stare at the priests' discolored or deformed hands during the blessing and thus put themselves in harm's way.

Tosefta (220 C.E.), commenting on this mishnah, expands on it and, simultaneously, mitigates its severity without exposing the congregation to the lethal holiness associated with the priestly blessing:

> A priest who has a blemish on his face, hands, or feet, lo this one should not raise his hands [in the priestly blessing], because the people will stare at him. But if he was an associate of the town [and therefore well known,] lo, this is permitted. (T. Megillah 3:29)

Tosefta first expands the teaching of the Mishnah. Not only should a priest with blemished hands not bless the congregation, but also one with blemished feet or face likewise should not come forward to recite the priestly benediction. The priests' feet would be visible to the congregation since their shoes are removed prior to giving the blessing. Somehow, too, the priests' faces must have been visible to the congregation at this ritual moment. Therefore, blemishes in any of these areas might cause congregants to stare at the priest and this could not be allowed. However, if many of the people worked in dyes, for example, so that the sight of someone with bright blue or red hands would not cause staring, or if the priest and his deformities were well-known to everyone and would likewise not engender extended gazing in his direction, then this priest represents no danger to the congregation and he may offer up the priestly benediction.

The Yerushalmi (400 C.E.) reports cases where these rules were applied selectively:

> Rabbi Naftali had crooked fingers. He came and asked Rabbi Mana [if he might offer the priestly blessing]. He [Rabbi Mana] said to him, "Since you are well known in your town it is permitted."
> Rav Huna would take away [someone with] a thin beard [from saying the priestly benediction]. But it was taught, "If he was well known in his city he is permitted [to recite the priestly blessing]." (Y. Megillah 4:8, 75b-c//Y. Taanit 4:1, 67b)

The Bavli (500 C.E.) upholds Tosefta's and the Yerushalmi's stance that, as long as a priest's blemish is familiar to the congregants and, we may infer, does not cause them to stare, then he is permitted to offer up the blessing.

> A tanna stated: The blemishes which [the sages] said [disqualify a priest] are on [the priest's] face, on his hands and on his feet.
> Rabbi Yehoshua ben Levi said: [If] his hands are spotted he should not lift up his hands [in the priestly blessing]. It has been taught similarly: If his hands are spotted, he should not lift up his hands. If they are curved inwards or bent sideways, he should not lift up his hands [in the priestly blessing]. . . .
> Rav Huna said: A man whose eyes run should not lift up his hands [in the priestly blessing]. But was there not one [such priest] in Rav Huna's neighborhood who used to spread forth his hands? [This was permitted because] he [was a resident] of the town [and his neighbors] were used to his appearance. It has been taught similarly: "A man whose eyes run should not lift up his hands [in the priestly blessing], but if he [was a resident] of the town [and his neighbors] were used to his appearance [and would not stare when he offered the blessing] he is permitted [to offer the blessing]."
> Rabbi Yochanan said: A [priest] blind in one eye should not lift up his hands [to offer the blessing]. But was there not one [such priest] in Rabbi Yochanan's neighborhood who used to spread forth his hands? He [was a resident] of the town [and his neighbors] were used to his appearance. It was taught similarly: "A man blind in one eye should not lift up his hands, but if the townspeople are

accustomed to him, he is permitted."

Rabbi Yehudah says: A man whose hands are discolored should not lift up his hands. . . . . [But] if most of the men of the town [work in] the same occupation it is permitted [since the off-color hands will not cause the congregation to stare]. (B. Megillah 24b)

The trend in these documents seems to tend toward ever-more lenient rulings allowing priests who are physically blemished to participate in the priestly blessing in the synagogue setting.

THE STUBBORN AND REBELLIOUS SON: MISUNDERSTANDING RESTRICTIONS

One of the harshest passages in Biblical literature is the one regarding the "stubborn and rebellious son":

If a man has a stubborn and rebellious son who does not listen to his father's voice or to his mother's voice, and they shall chasten him and he [still] will not listen to them. [Then] his father and his mother will lay hold of him and take him out to the elders of his city and to the gate of his place. And they shall say to the elders of his city, "This, our son, is stubborn and rebellious and will not listen to our voice. He is a glutton and a drunkard." And all the people of his city shall stone him with stones and he shall die. And you shall put out evil from among you and all Israel shall hear [of it] and fear. (Deuteronomy 21:18-21)

The sages abhorred the death penalty and used every means to make it almost impossible to administer capital punishment. (Indeed, T. Sanhedrin 11:6 states that there never was, nor will there ever be, a stubborn and rebellious son.) It was for this reason that they interpreted the Biblical passage, above, in a way that appears to discriminate against those with disabilities.

If one of them [the parents of a stubborn, rebellious son] had a maimed hand, or was lame, or was blind, or was mute or was deaf, he [their son] cannot be made a stubborn and rebellious son. For it is said, "And his father and his mother shall lay hold of him (Deuteronomy 21:19)" and [those] with maimed hands cannot [do so].

"And bring him out (Deuteronomy 21:19)" and [those who are] lame cannot [do so]. "And they shall say (Deuteronomy 21:20)" and [those who are] mute cannot [do so]. "This, our son (Deuteronomy 21:20)" and [those who are] blind cannot [do so because the phrase implies they are pointing to the son]. "He does not hearken to our voice (Deuteronomy 21:20)" and [those who are] deaf cannot [hear whether their son has listened to them or not]. (M. Sanhredrin 8:4//Sifre D. Piska 219)

In interpreting the passage in this way, the sages make the requirements for testimony in this case almost as stringent as the qualifications for officiating in the priesthood. However, they do so solely to legislate this punishment out of existence by limiting it through any means possible. After all, having a hand has no logical effect on one's ability to give cogent testimony and, indeed, nothing bars a person with a maimed hand from testifying in any other matter. It is only in this case that the sages make such a ruling. Understanding their motivation correctly allows us to see that their aim was not to discriminate against those with disabilities but to minimize the number of executions of "stubborn and rebellious" sons.

ISRAEL DISABLED

In the powerful prophetic image of Isaiah's suffering servant (52:13-53:5) we find an explicit linking of sin, disabilities, suffering and atonement. The suffering servant is clearly disabled and wounded. His wounds, like the sacrifices in the Temple, make expiation for sin:

Behold, my servant shall prosper, he shall be exalted and extolled, and be very high. As many were astonished at you, saying, Surely his visage is too marred to be human, and his form, to be from humanity ['s mold] so shall he startle many nations. Kings shall shut their mouths: for that which they had not been told them shall they see; and that which they had not heard they shall comprehend. Who [would have] believed our report and to whom is the arm of God's arm revealed? For he grew up before him as a tender plant, and as a root out of a dry ground: he had no form or comeliness, that we should look at him, and no countenance, that we should desire him. He was [the most] despised and rejected of men; a man of pains, and knowing sickness: and we hid (as it were) our faces from him; he was despised, and we considered him not. But he has borne our sicknesses and endured our pains; yet we considered him stricken, smitten of God, and afflicted. But he was wounded because of our transgressions, bruised because of our iniquities: his sufferings were that we might have peace, and by his injury we are healed. (Isaiah 52:13-53:5)

The Suffering Servant appears in Deutero-Isaiah, i.e., the author of Isaiah chapters 40-55 who lived in Babylonia during the exile and wrote during the sixth century B.C.E. The Suffering Servant, then, is the literary creation of a stateless teacher, trying to define Judaism in exile. He has no role in politics, war or the cult. Rather, it is through his devotion in the face of suffering that he attains his purpose. This description could also fit the situation of the sages after 70 C.E. Significantly, it is the sages who will later emphasize this concept, that suffering may replace the atonement previously found in the cult.

Israel is sometimes characterized metaphorically as a person with a disability. Here, the use of one gestalt to explain another is obvious: moral disability > physical disability. Israel is conceived of as a person's body and her immorality is symbolized by physical disabilities. Isaiah characterizes Israel as willfully disabling herself:

Hear, deaf ones and look [in order] to see, blind ones! Who is blind but my servant or deaf, as my messenger whom I sent? Who is blind as the one I send, and blind as God's servant? Seeing much but observing nothing; [having] hearing hears but not attending. (Isaiah 42:18-20)

Israel's deafness and blindness are not due to any lack of properly functioning organs. It is specifically stated: God's servants have eyes and ears which presumably operate but they are too stubborn and willful to see and understand the truth of God's message with those organs. When they stop being recalcitrant, and "blinding themselves" to the reality of God's presence, they will, themselves, become the "light of the world":

I, God, have called you in righteousness, and will hold your hand, and will keep you, and place you [as] a covenant people, [as] a light for the nations; to open the blind eyes, to bring out the prisoners from the prison, and them that sit in darkness out of the prison house. (Isaiah 42:6-7)

In this passage, the "blind eye" is clearly meant as a metaphor for bringing knowledge of God to those who lack it rather than physical blindness. Sight, once more, stands for insight.

Yet, for the sages, outward beauty is far from the sign of inward grace. Indeed, they envision the messiah as a person with disabilities:

> What is the [identifying] mark [of the messiah]? He sits among the poor, those suffering disease. And they all take off their bandages at one time and put them back on at one time. But he [the messiah] takes off one bandage at a time and puts it back on, saying: Perhaps I will be needed and I do not want to be delayed. (B. Sanhedrin 98a)

This vision of the messiah is almost the photo-negative of the image of the priest in the Torah. The messiah is ritually impure (the disease, it is inferred, is leprosy which makes one ritually impure), excluded from society, sitting outside one of the city's gates while the priests are allowed inside God's sanctuary. Though physically blemished and ritually impure, this is the one through whom redemption will come.

doi: 10.1300/J095v10n03_06

What the Rabbis Heard:
Deafness in the *Mishnah*

Bonnie L. Gracer, MA, MSW

SUMMARY. This article examines deafness in Jewish antiquity as expressed in the *Mishnah*, the foundation document of rabbinic Judaism. Ancient Greek and Roman attitudes towards disability and deafness are surveyed in order to establish the context within which the *Mishnah* was formulated, and to assess whether, and to what extent, Greco-Roman beliefs may have influenced the rabbis and Jewish law on matters pertaining to deafness. Particular focus is given to (a) infanticide and gratitude and two opposing responses to disability in antiquity; and (b) the common belief the hearing and speech are precursors to intelligence. The major findings of this article are that while the rabbis of the *Mishnah* did not adopt the Greco-Roman practice of infanticide in response to the

---

The research for this article began in partial fulfillment of the requirements for the author's master's degree in Jewish Studies, with an emphasis on Ancient Judaism, at Baltimore Hebrew University. The author gratefully acknowledges and thanks Professor Steven Fine, then of Baltimore Hebrew University, now at the University of Cincinnati, Professor Cheryl Walker of Brandeis University, the late Professor Irving Kenneth Zola (z"l) of Brandeis University, and Rabbi Jonathan Kraus of Belmont, Massachusetts for their teaching, inspiration, and assistance. All honor is due them. All errors are the author's.

Queries to the author or responses to the article can be directed through the Co-Editor of this collection, Bill Gaventa (E-mail: gaventwi@umdnj.edu).

Reprinted with permission from *Disabilities Studies Quarterly* from its Spring 2003 Issue. Volume 23, Number 2 <www.dsq-sds.org>.

[Haworth co-indexing entry note]: "What the Rabbis Heard: Deafness in the *Mishnah*." Gracer, Bonnie L. Co-published simultaneously in *Journal of Religion, Disability & Health* (The Haworth Pastoral Press, an imprint of The Haworth Press, Inc.) Vol. 10, No. 3/4, 2006, pp. 85-99; and: *Jewish Perspectives on Theology and the Human Experience of Disability* (ed: Rabbi Judith Z. Abrams, and William C. Gaventa) The Haworth Pastoral Press, an imprint of The Haworth Press, Inc., 2006, pp. 85-99. Single or multiple copies of this article are available for a fee from The Haworth Document Delivery Service [1-800-HAWORTH, 9:00 a.m. - 5:00 p.m. (EST). E-mail address: docdelivery@haworthpress.com].

Available online at http://jrdh.haworthpress.com

doi:10.1300/J095v10n03_07

birth of a child with a disability, they did incorporate beliefs about the connections between hearing, speech, and intelligence into Jewish law. This article surveys the *Mishnah* in order to elaborate on these points and discuss their implications for the participation of deaf people in Jewish life. doi:10.1300/J095v10n03_07 *[Article copies available for a fee from The Haworth Document Delivery Service: 1-800-HAWORTH. E-mail address: <docdelivery@haworthpress.com> Website: <http://www.HaworthPress.com>]*

KEYWORDS. Judaism, deafness, disability, antiquity, *Mishnah*, halacha, Ancient Greece and Rome

INTRODUCTION

This article examines deafness in Jewish antiquity as expressed in the *Mishnah*,[1] the foundation document of rabbinic Judaism. Ancient Greek and Roman attitudes towards disability and deafness are surveyed in order to establish the context within which the *Mishnah* was formulated, and to assess whether, and to what extent, Greco-Roman beliefs may have influenced the rabbis and Jewish law on matters pertaining to deafness. Particular focus is given to (a) infanticide and gratitude as two opposing responses to disability in antiquity; and (b) the common belief that hearing and speech are precursors to intelligence. The major findings of this article are that while the rabbis of the *Mishnah* did not adopt the Greco-Roman practice of infanticide in response to the birth of a child with a disability, they did incorporate Greco-Roman beliefs about the connections between hearing, speech, and intelligence into Jewish law. This article surveys the *Mishnah* in order to elaborate on these points and discuss their implications for the participation of deaf people in Jewish life.

DISABILITY: A TIME TO KILL, A TIME TO BLESS

This section explores two distinct responses to disability in ancient times: murder, and gratitude.

Ancient Greece and Rome

In ancient Greece, infanticide was an accepted response to the birth of a child with a disability. Hippocrates raised the question, "which children should be raised?"[2] The responses of Plato (c. 427-347 B.C.E.) and Aristotle (c. 384-322 B.C.E.) make clear that people with disabilities were not among those slated to live. Plato stated, for example:

> This then is the kind of medical and judicial provision for which you will legislate in your state. It will provide treatment for those of your citizens whose physical and psychological constitution is good; as for the others, it will leave the unhealthy to die, and those whose psychological constitution is incurably corrupt it will put to death. That seems to be the best thing for both the individual sufferer and for society.[3]

Aristotle was in full agreement: "With regard to the choice between abandoning an infant or rearing it, let there be a law that no crippled child be reared."[4] Plato and Plutarch go so far as to provide detail on the process of making the decision about who should live and who should die. Plato stated: ". . . we must look at our offspring from every angle to make sure we are not taken in by a lifeless phantom not worth the rearing."[5] Plutarch maintained that the decision lay with the tribal elders rather than with the father.[6] The mother, apparently, was not part of the decision-making process.

In Rome (c. 450-449 B.C.E.), contemporary Roman custom was codified in a legal document known as the Twelve Tables. Lewis and Reinhold (1990) note that although certain parts of the Twelve Tables became antiquated, they never were repealed. They remained, at least in theory, the foundation of Roman law for the next 1000 years.[7] The Twelve Tables granted the male head of the family (the *paterfamilias*) exclusive power over his sons and daughters, including power over life and death.[8] Table IV of the Twelve Tables states: "kill quickly. . . a dreadfully deformed child."[9] The life and death power of the *paterfamilias* disappeared by the second century C.E., and by the third century C.E., abandoning a child was considered murder.[10]

Ancient Judaism

In contrast to the evidence of infanticide as a response to disability in ancient Greece and Rome, the *Mishnah* records no debates on whether people with disabilities should be allowed to live; infanticide is never even raised as a possibility. Quite the contrary–the rabbis cherish life and see human variety as evidence of God's greatness. This is evident in the *Mishnah* and later rabbinic literature. For example, *M. Sanhedrin* 4:5 states:

... whoever destroys a single soul ..., Scripture accounts it as if he had destroyed a full world; and whoever saves one soul ..., Scripture accounts it as if he had saved a full world ... declare the greatness of the Holy One ... for man stamps out many coins with one die, and they are all alike, but the King of Kings, the Holy One ... stamped each man with the seal of Adam, and not one of them is like his fellow.[11]

The *Mishnah* also states: "One is obliged to bless for the evil—just as one blesses for the good ... Whatever treatment God metes out to you, thank Him very, very much."[12] Moses Maimonides (1135–1204) later explains (in his commentary on this *Mishnah)*: "There are many things that seem good initially, but turn out evil in the end. Hence the wise man is not confounded when great troubles befall him, since he does not know what will eventuate."[13]

But how does all of this relate to disability? Other than not killing children with disabilities, how is society to respond, according to the *Tannaim*,[14] the rabbis of the Mishnah? They are to respond with gratitude and blessing. This is evident in two blessings of rabbinic origin: the "True Judge" blessing and the "varied creatures" blessing. *M. Brachot* 9:2 directs: "On hearing bad tidings, (one) says: 'Blessed is the True Judge.' " The Tosefta[15] clarifies the application of this blessing to disability: "[One who sees] an amputee, or a lame person, or a blind person, or a person afflicted with boils, says, 'Blessed [are you Lord our God, Ruler of the Universe], the True Judge.' "[16] As for varied creatures, the Tosefta also directs:

One who sees an Ethiopian, or an albino, or a [man] red-spotted in the face, or [a man] white spotted in the face, or a hunchback, or a dwarf (or a *cheresh* or a *shoteh* or a drunk person) says, "Blessed [are you Lord our God, Ruler of the Universe who creates such] varied creatures.[17]

The Jerusalem Talmud, a later rabbinic elaboration on the *Mishnah,* discusses the differences between the "True Judge" and "varied creatures" blessings:

This teaching [to say the blessing, 'the True Judge'] applies [to those who see persons with disabilities who were born] whole and later were changed. But if [one sees a person who] was born that way he says, 'Blessed [are you Lord our God, Ruler of the Universe who creates such] varied creatures."[18]

Judith Abrams concludes, "If one is born without disabilities and they later develop, then the disabilities are a judgement from God. Those born with disabilities, however, are simply among God's varied creatures."[19] In either case, it is evident that both the *Tannaim* and the later rabbis considered encountering persons with disabilities as occasions to bless and thank God, not as occasions to kill.

SPEECH, HEARING, AND INTELLIGENCE

Oral debate and dialogue were core activities at the heart of the ancient world. In the Greco-Roman world, this was manifest, for example, in Plato's Socratic Dialogues (and the Socratic method of teaching by questioning), in the emphasis on both tragic and comic plays,[20] and in the speeches, debate and discussion in the Roman Senate. In ancient Judaism, rabbinic law was passed down from one generation to the next by means of oral and aural transmission of knowledge. Indeed, *"Torah sh'be-al peh"*–Torah from the mouth, or Oral Torah[21]–transformed Judaism from a biblical to a rabbinic religion.

Words were critical to ancient society.[22] What, then, did the ancients understand about deafness and deaf people?

Ancient Greece and Rome

Martha Edwards, in her extensive discussion of disability in ancient Greece, notes:

> Language was the hallmark of human achievement, so muteness went beyond a physical condition. An inability to speak went hand-in-hand with an inability to reason, hand-in-hand with stupidity. Plato (*Theaetetus* 206d) has Socrates say that anyone can show what he thinks about anything, unless he is speechless or deaf from birth.[23]

Aristotle made profound connections between hearing, speech, and intelligence.[24] In a statement that was to have profound implications for the education of deaf individuals henceforth, Aristotle stated:

> . . . it is hearing that contributes most to the growth of intelligence. For rational discourse is a cause of instruction in virtue of its being audible . . . Accordingly, of persons destitute from birth of either sense, the blind are more intelligent than the deaf and dumb.[25]

Aristotle also asserted that "Men that are born deaf are in all cases also dumb;[26] that is, they can make vocal sounds, but they cannot speak."[27] Benderly, describing this statement as "widely mistranslated," notes that: " Because many took 'speechless' to mean 'stupid,' the authority whose word ruled Western thought for over a thousand years appeared to state that the congenitally deaf were necessarily congenital morons."[28]

The passionate emotion in Benderly's writing is common in the history of deafness–and no wonder. The link between hearing, speech, intelligence, and the ability to learn has had staggering educational consequences.[29] Radutsky reports, for example,

> . . . the Romans did not consider deafness a separate phenomenon
> from mutism and . . . consequently, many believed all deaf people
> were incapable of being educated. Ancient Roman law, in fact,
> classified deaf people as *'mentecatti furiosi'*–which may be trans-
> lated roughly as raving maniacs–and claimed them uneducable.[30]

The Roman writer Pliny the Elder (23-79 C.E.), in *Natural History*, writes: "there are no persons born deaf who are not also dumb."[31] As Benderly has noted, confusion over the terms "dumb," "stupid," and "mute" has had serious repercussions for deaf people throughout history.

Ancient Judaism

The *Tannaim* appear to have incorporated Aristotelian connections between hearing, speech, and intelligence into Jewish tradition. The *Mishnah* sets forth two types of categories through which to examine deafness. The first is a larger category, into which deaf people fit, and the second is a series of smaller, more deafness-specific categories. The larger category is grouped as *"cheresh, shoteh ve-katan"*–"a deaf-mute, a mentally defective person, and a minor." This category is noteworthy in its apparent linking of deafness and muteness[32] with cognitive abilities and moral reasoning. The more specific categories include: "deaf mute";[33] "deaf and can speak";[34] one who has "become a deaf-mute";[35] a "deaf-mute who recovered his senses";[36] a "deaf-mute" who "recovered his speech";[37] and "deaf."[38] These categories are noteworthy in two respects. First, their focus on "senses" and speech suggests parallels to Aristotelian thought and demonstrates the importance of hearing and speech to the *Tannaim*. Second, the categories demonstrate a recognition of human difference–including differing abilities and modes of communication in deaf people.

The major concern of the rabbis seems to have been whether a deaf person (*cheresh*) could develop *da'at*–knowledge, intelligence, morality, reasoning abilities.[39] It is here that Aristotle's pronouncements regarding the connections between speech, hearing, and intelligence seem to be paralleled: voice is connected to soul and imagination; audition is connected to rational discourse; hearing is connected to intelligence.

Both with respect to participation in society and responsibility for wrongdoing, these beliefs had serious, real-life consequences. On the one hand, social and religious opportunities were limited for deaf people. *M. Arachin* 1:1 states, for example, ". . . a deaf-mute, a mentally defective person, and a minor" may not vow or dedicate the worth of another, because they possess no understanding (*da'at*) (to formulate vows nor to make assessments) (italics mine). On the other hand, deaf people appear to have been treated leniently with respect to criminal justice situations. For example, the *Mishnah* describes situations where able-bodied persons were held responsible and punished for damage or wrongdoing, but deaf persons were not. *M. Baba Kamma* 8:4 states, "It is a bad thing [for anyone] to knock against a deaf-mute, a mentally defective person, or a minor, since he that wounds them is liable, whereas if they wound others they are not liable." And according to *M. Baba Kama* 4:4,

> If an ox of a person of sound senses gored an ox of a deaf-mute, or a mentally-defective person, or a minor, he is liable; but if one belonging to a deaf-mute, or a mentally-defective person, or a minor gored an ox of one of sound senses, he is exempt.

Deaf people, it seems, could injure others (or let their animals injure others) and get away with it.[40] Why? The rabbis, like Aristotle, seem to have linked deafness with some sort of moral or cognitive deficiency. Rabbinic pedagogy relied heavily on verbal communication. Prime activities included verbal arguing, discussing, and questioning. Without the ability to participate in the discussions and arguments, deaf people may have been seen as having no way to develop or communicate *halachic* or other reasoning skills.[41]

The link between deafness (*cheresh*) and intelligence/understanding (*da'at*) for the rabbis, as for Aristotle, appears to have been speech. *M. Terumoth* 1:1 and 1:2, when examined together, illuminate this point. *M. Terumoth* 1:1 states,

There are five who *may not* separate the priest's share of the produce, and if they do so their separation *is not* valid . . . a deaf-mute (*cheresh*), an insane person (*shoteh*), and a minor (*katan*) . . . (parentheses and underlines mine).[42]

Compare this to *M. Terumoth* 1:2:

A deaf person–such as can speak but can not hear (*cheresh ha-m'daber v'aino shomayah lo*)–should not separate . . . but if he did so his separated priest's share is valid (parentheses and underlines mine).

In *M. Terumoth* 1:1, the *cheresh* has no chance of his separation being valid. In *M. Terumoth* 1:2, he does. The *cheresh* in 1:1 "may not" separate. The *cheresh* in 1:2 "should not" separate. Legally, this may have been a major distinction. In 1:1, if a *cheresh* separated anyway the separation still was not valid. In 1:2 it was. And what was the only difference between the deaf people in the two Mishnaic traditions? Speech. As if to answer any remaining question, *M. Terumoth* 1:2 continues: "The *cheresh* of whom the Sages have spoken in all cases is one who can neither hear nor speak."

Even without the linking of hearing and intelligence, the simple ability to hear and speak clearly had important implications for participation and leadership in rabbinic society. Take, for example, the religious obligation to recite the *"Shema,"* a defining prayer in the Jewish liturgy. The Hebrew word *"Shema"* typically is translated as "hear." The first line of the prayer reads: "Hear O Israel, the Lord is our God, the Lord is One."[43] The *Mishnah* records the following debate:

If someone read the *Shema* but did not hear it, he fulfills his obligation. Rabbi Yose said, He has not fulfilled his obligation.[44]

Pinchas Kehati (a recent commentator), noting that "R. Yose's ruling is the norm," explains: "[He has not fulfilled his obligation] . . . to read the *Shema*, since the verse reads, 'Hear. . . ' make audible to your ear what your mouth has to say (*Gemara*)." However, it is worth noting that an alternate translation of the word *"shema"* is "understand." The first *Tanna*, Kehati explains, "interprets S*hema* to mean 'understand' (as in II Kings 18:26-tr), hence, 'S*hema*–In any language that you understand.' It is permissible, then, for one to recite the *Shema* in any language he understands."[45] The *mishnah* continues:

If one read the *Shema* without enunciating the letters properly, R. Yose says, He has fulfilled his obligation. Rabbi Yehudah says, He has not fulfilled his obligation.[46]

In this instance R. Yose's ruling also prevails. However, Kehati notes that ". . . *ab initio* one is required to pronounce the letters precisely and to take care not to run two identical or similar letters into one . . . "[47] While people with hearing and/or speech impairments are not explicitly discussed in this *mishnah*, questions certainly arise: can a deaf person who cannot hear or speak clearly fulfill the obligation to recite the S*hema?* Could the anonymous Mishnah's interpretation of "*shema*" as "understand" rather than "hear" mean a deaf person could fulfill the obligation by reciting the prayer in sign language, if that is a language he or she understands? These are questions of Jewish law best examined in a separate venue;[48] for now, it is worthwhile simply to note the importance of hearing and speech to the rabbis of the *Mishnah*.

Similarly, the Rosh Hashanah liturgy requires Jews to "hear the sound of the *shofar*."[49] The *Mishnaic* tractate on Rosh Hashanah states, "A deaf-mute, an imbecile, and a minor cannot fulfill an obligation on behalf of the many. This is the general rule: whoever is not liable to an obligation, cannot fulfill that obligation on behalf of the many."[50] Kehati offers the following commentary:

> Resuming the discussion of fulfilling the obligation of blowing the *shofar* on behalf of others, the *mishnah* teaches that a person can do so only if he himself is liable to that obligation. A deaf-mute, an imbecile . . . and a minor . . . are not liable to the commandment of the *shofar*, and therefore they cannot fulfill an obligation on behalf of the many . . . According to one opinion, a person who is deaf but can speak may also not fulfill this obligation on behalf of others, for the essence of the commandment is "to hear the sound of the *shofar*," and since he does not hear, he is exempt.[51]

Finally, *Tannatic* rulings demonstrate an impressive awareness of deafness-specific issues. For example, the existence of a separate category for an individual who had "become a deaf-mute"[52] suggests an understanding of age-of-onset (of deafness) as a critical factor in speech and language development. And it is clear that the *Tannaim* understood that deaf people communicated both manually and orally. For example, *M. Gittin* (5:7) states, "A deaf-mute (*cheresh*) may transact business by signs and be communicated with by signs"–and then continues, "Ben

Bathyra says, he may transact business and be communicated with by lip movements in matters concerning movable property." And *M. Yevamot* (14:1) states, "Just as he marries by gesture so he may divorce by gesture."[53] The nature of these activities (marriage, divorce, business dealings) requires intelligence, reason, and knowledge–*da'at*. So perhaps the rabbis (at least some of them, some of the time) understood that meaningful, abstract concepts (as well as detail) could be communicated manually, and that deaf people might have some access to *da'at*.

CONCLUSION

The Jewish Bible, known in Hebrew as the *Torah,* was the basis of the rabbinic discussion and exegesis that led to the development of the *Mishnah* and later Jewish law. And so it is perhaps fitting to end this article with a story from *Torah*–the story of the great leader and prophet Moses, who had a speech impairment. According to the Book of Exodus, God commanded Moses to free the Israelites from slavery in Egypt. Moses, however, hesitated: "Please, O Lord, I have never been a man of words. I am slow of speech and slow of tongue." God responded, "Who gives man speech? Who makes him dumb or deaf or seeing or blind? Is it not I, the Lord? Now go, and I will be with you as you speak . . . " Still, Moses protested: "Please, O Lord, make someone else Your agent."[54] And then, in what I can describe only as the first reasonable accommodation in the *Torah*, God assured Moses that Aaron, his brother, who "speaks readily"–would join him and speak for him.[55] And with that, Moses helped form a band of former slaves into a new nation, witnessed revelation, and delivered to the world the Ten Commandments.[56] Whatever one believes about the origin, truth, or veracity of the biblical text, the *Torah* demonstrates, through the story of Moses, the enormous potential of each human being. Moses should have been killed when he was an infant–Pharaoh had decreed the murder of all newborn Hebrew boys, and Moses was one. Imagine the implications.

Given the central role of *Torah* in *Mishnaic* and later Jewish law and tradition, it is not surprising that the *Mishnah* credits a person who saves a single soul with having saved a whole world.[57] It is not surprising that the *Mishnah* does not decree (or even contemplate) the murder of children with (or without) disabilities. It makes sense that the *Mishnah* is able to envision alternative means of communication for people who are deaf or who have speech impairments.

At the same time, the ancient Jews did live amongst the ancient Greeks and Romans. It is therefore not surprising that the rabbis, as evidenced in the *Mishnaic* canon, incorporated into Jewish law Greco-Roman beliefs linking hearing, speech, intelligence, and morality. It is clear, however, that the rabbis viewed all people, including deaf people, as unique individuals. The Mishnaic delineation of multiple categories of deafness resulted in not *every* deaf person being "categorically" disqualified or exempt from the performance of specific *mitzvot*.[58] The rabbis observed deaf people, paid enough attention to notice detail, and deemed deaf people worthy of life, legal rulings, and protections. From the standpoint of deaf history, these are all extremely positive developments.

NOTES

1. The *Mishnah* documents the debates, rulings, and sayings of the *Tannaim,* five generations of rabbis who lived c. 50 B.C.E. through 200 C.E. A whole body of literature and legislation developed from the text of the *Mishnah.* Generations of rabbis (known as the *Amoraim* and *Savoraim,* c. 200-700 CE), debated and analyzed the *Mishnaic* canon and from it, further developed Jewish law. The debates and discussions of the *Amoraim* and *Savoraim* are embodied in the *Babylonian Talmud.* Judaism continued to develop, with each successive generation studying the *Mishnah, Talmud,* and ensuing rabbinic works, and applying them to the issues of their day. The *Mishnah* consists of 63 tractates, or sections, and covers a broad array of topics such as ethics, civil law, damages, agriculture, holidays, women, children, marriage, divorce, religious ritual, and Jewish liturgy. Discussions of disability and deafness are scattered throughout; therefore, the examples in this article are given in the context of a variety of issues. For a survey of Rabbinic literature and introduction of its constituent documents, see Strack and Stemberger, 1996. On the *Mishnah,* pp. 108-148.

2. As quoted in Winzer (1997:82).

3. *The Republic,* Book III, 409e-410a.

4. *Politics,* 7, 1335b., 19-21.

5. *Theaetetus* (160E-161A), as quoted in Martha L. Edwards (1996:82).

6. *Plutarch's Lives*, Vol. I., Lycurgus, 16.

7. Lewis and Reinhold (1990:107-8) also note that Cicero (106 B.C.E.- 43 C.E.) reported that in his time, boys were required to memorize the Twelve Tables (*Laws* II. xxiii. 59).

8. Casson (1998:10-11), noting that infanticide was practiced throughout ancient times, adds that the decisions of the *paterfamilias* were made "not necessarily in consultation with the mother." Casson (1998: 10-11) also notes other reasons for infanticide, such as poverty (on the one hand), and the division of property amongst too many heirs (on the other). Carcopino (1968:77) adds that girl babies and "bastards" were victims of exposure.

9. Lewis and Reinhold (1990: 110). The Twelve Tables were instituted as a means of plebian protection against patrician magistrates, and as a means of equality before the law.

10. Carcopino (1968:77).

11. Individual sayings, laws, and discussions within the *Mishnah* also are called mishnahs, and are cited according to Tractate. For example, the *mishnah* quoted above is located in chapter four of Tractate *Sanhedrin*. Its citation reads "*M. Sanhedrin* 4:5" because it is the fifth *mishnah* in chapter four of Tractate *Sanhedrin*.

12. *M. Berakhot* 9:5.

13. Kehati commentary to *M. Berakhot 9:5*.

14. The term *"Tannaim"* refers to five generations of rabbis who lived c. 50 B.C.E. to 200 C.E., whose debates, rulings, and sayings are documented in the *Mishnah*.

15. The *Tosefta* is a compilation of *Tannaitic* sayings not included in the *Mishnaic* canon. See Strack and Stemberger, pp. 149-163.

16. *T. Berakhot* 6:3. Translation follows Judith Abrams (1998:118).

17. *T. Berakhot* 6:3. Translation follows Judith Abrams (1998:118-19).

18. *Y. Berakhot* 9:1. Translation follows Judith Abrams (1998:119). On the Jerusalem Talmud, Strack and Stemberger, 164-189.

19. Judith Abrams (1998:119).

20. e.g., Euripides, Aristophanes, Sophocles, Aeschylus.

21. "Oral Torah" refers to the belief that Moses received two Torahs on Mt. Sinai—one written, one oral. The basis for this belief is in *M. Avot* 1:1, and is extrapolated in part from the appearance of the plural *"Torot"* in *Leviticus* 26:46. The phrase in Leviticus reads, "These are the decrees, the ordinances, and the teachings (*Torot*) that God gave, between Himself and the Children of Israel, at Mount Sinai, through Moses." *"Torot"* is plural of the word *"Torah,"* suggesting that two Torahs were given to Moses. The rabbis explained that the first *Torah* was the written one (*Torah she-bi-ktav*), and the second was the oral one. For further discussion, see Elon (1994:190-227), Safrai (1987:35-120), and Shiffman (1991:177-200).

22. Boman, discussing the origins of the Greek *"logos"* (word), notes, "*Logos*, word, came from . . . 'to speak.' The basic meaning of the root *leg-* is, without doubt, 'to gather' . . . to put together in order, *to arrange* . . . The deepest level of meaning in the term 'word' is thus nothing which has to do with the function of speaking—neither dynamic spokeness . . . nor the articulateness of utterance—but the meaning, the ordered and reasonable content . . . *Logos* expresses the mental function that is highest according to Greek understanding," Boman (1970:67).

23. Martha Edwards (1995). Physical Disability in the Ancient Greek World. UMI Dissertation Services, p. 101.

24. In *On the Soul*, Book II, 420b.5, and 420b.29-421a.1, Aristotle also said that the soul resides in the windpipe and the areas of the body that create speech, and that "voice is sound with a meaning."

25. *Sense and Sensibilia*, 436b.16-437a.15.

26. Benderly (1980:107) translates "dumb" as "speechless."

27. *History of Animals*, Book IV, 9, 536b.4.

28. Benderly (1980:107).

29. Ancient ideas of speech as an indicator of intelligence set the stage for what later became a communications debate so passionate that Benderly called it "a holy war . . . a conflict as fierce as any that ever sundered a party cell or shattered a religious denomi-

nation." Known initially as the "War of Methods" and later as the "oral/manual controversy," the debate focused on whether deaf people should communicate by speaking or signing (Brill, 1984:17, Benderly, 1980:vii-8, Lane, 1984, Lane and Phillips, 1984), Spradley and Spradley, 1978), Winefield, 1987).

30. Radutsky, 1993:239. Pliny (*Natural History* 35,21), however, does record a celebrated debate when the grandson of Quintus Pedius, a former consul who was appointed by Caesar as his joint heir with Augustus, was born *mutus*. Both Augustus and the orator Messala agreed that the grandson, also named Quintus Pedius, should have lessons in painting. Apparently the child made great progress before he died at an early age.

31. As cited in Wright, 1969:136, and Benderly, 1980:107.

32. The cochlea, inner ear and mechanisms of hearing actually have no direct bearing on the vocal chords or the ability to speak. The reason "deaf speech" sounds different is that deaf people cannot hear how sounds are pronounced.

33. *M. Terumoth* 1:1.

34. *M. Terumoth* 1:2.

35. *M. Yevamoth* 14:1; *M. Sotah* 4:5.

36. *M. Gittin* 2:6.

37. *M. Baba Kamma* 4:4.

38. *M. Sanhedrin* 8:4.

39. Abrams, 1998.

40. See also *M. Sanhedrin* 8:4, in which hearing children of deaf adults also appear to be treated leniently.

41. "*Halachah*" means Jewish law.

42. The "separation" under discussion is the Heave-offering (*terumah*)–the portion of one's harvest that must be given to the priests in the Temple before one can eat from one's harvest. The remaining two who may not separate are "he who separates the *priest's-due* from that which is not his own, and a non-Jew who separated from that of a Jew even by permission."

43. This prayer comes from *Deuteronomy* 6:4, and articulates the Jewish belief in one God.

44. *M. Berakhot* 2:3.

45. Kehati on *M. Berakhot* 2:3. "*Tanna*" is the singular form of the Hebrew word "*Tannaim.*"

46. *M. Berakhot* 2:3.

47. Kehati on *M. Berakhot* 2:3.

48. For a more current discussion of Jewish law and deafness, for example, see Mordechai Shuchatowitz's "Halacha Concerning Jewish Deaf and Hard of Hearing" published by the Orthodox Union (undated).

49. A *shofar* is a ram's horn. When blown, it creates a loud sound. For a survey of the Jewish holidays, including Rosh Hashana, see Greenberg (1988).

50. *M. Rosh Hashanah* 3:8.

51. Kehati commentary on *M. Rosh Hashana* 3:8.

52. *M. Yevamoth* 14:1, *M. Sotah* 4:5.

53. Blackman (1963) alternately translates "sign" (*M. Gittin* 5:7), and "gesture" (*M. Yevamot* 14:1). The Hebrew in both instances stems from the root letters *reish, mem, zayin*. Alcalay (1996:2462) defines this, in part, as "hint, imply, sign, gesture." Blackman defines it as "sign, deaf and dumb language" (see footnote to *M. Yevamot* 14:1).

54. *Exodus* 4:10-13.
55. *Exodus* 4:14-16.
56. The Book of *Exodus* details the life of Moses.
57. *M. Sanhedrin* 4:5.
58. *"Mitzvot"* is plural of *"mitzvah,"* a Hebrew word meaning "commandment."

REFERENCES

Abrams, Judith Z. (1998). *Judaism and Disability: Portrayals in Ancient Texts from the Tanach Through the Bavli.* Washington, DC: Gallaudet University Press.

Albeck, Chanoch (1952). *The Mishnah.* Jerusalem: Mosad Bialik (Hebrew.)

Alcalay, Reuben (1996). *The Complete Hebrew-English Dictionary.* Tel-Aviv: Miskal Publishing and Distribution, LTD.

Barnes, Jonathan (1984). *The Complete Works of Aristotle.* The Revised Oxford Translation. Vol. I, Bollinger Series LXXI.2. Princeton: Princeton University Press.

Benderly, Beryl Lieff (1980). *Dancing Without Music: Deafness in America.* Garden City: Anchor Press/Doubleday.

Blackman, Philip (1990). *Mishnayoth* (2nd ed.). Gateshead: Judaica Press, LTD.

Boman, Thorleif (1970). *Hebrew Thought Compared with Greek.* New York: Norton & Company.

Brill, Richard G. (1984). *International Congresses on the Education of the Deaf: An Analytical History (1878-1980).* Washington, DC: Gallaudet University Press.

Carcopino, Jerome (1960). *Daily Life in Ancient Rome: The People and the City at the Height of the Empire.* New Haven: Yale University Press.

Casson, Lionel (1998). *Everyday Life in Ancient Rome.* Baltimore: Johns Hopkins University Press.

Clough, Arthur Hugh (editor) (2001). *Lycurgus.* In *Plutarch's Lives*, Vol. 1. The Dryden Translation. New York: The Modern Library.

Edwards, Martha L. (1997). Deaf and Dumb in Ancient Greece. In L. J. Davis, *The Disability Studies Reader.* New York: Routledge.

Edwards, Martha L. (1996). 'Let There Be a Law that No Deformed Child Shall be Reared': The Cultural Context of Deformity in the Ancient Greek World. *The Ancient History Bulletin*, 10.3-4, 79-92.

Edwards, Martha L. (1995). Physical Disability in the Ancient Greek World. Unpublished Doctoral Dissertation, Ann Arbor: UMI Dissertation Services.

Elon, Menachem (1994). *Jewish Law: History, Sources, Principles.* Philadelphia: Jewish Publication Society.

Greenberg, Irving (1988). *The Jewish Way: Living the Holidays.* New York: Simon and Shuster.

Kahana, Nachman (Tr.) (undated). *Seder Zeraim: Berakhot.* A New Translation with a Commentary by Rabbi Pinchas Kehati. Jerusalem: Maor Wallach Press.

Kehati, Pinchas (1966-1977). *Mishnah.* Mishnavot mevo'arot/bi-yede Pinhas Kehati. (Hebrew.) Jerusalem: Hekhal Shelomoh.

Lane, Harlan (1984). *When the Mind Hears: A History of the Deaf*. New York: Random House.

Lee, Desmond (Tr.) (1987). *Plato: The Republic*. London: Penguin Classics.

Levin, Edward (Tr.) (1994). *Seder Moed: Mishnah Rosh Hashana, Mishnah Megilla: A New Translation with a Commentary by Rabbi Pinchas Kehati*. Jerusalem: Maor Wallach Press.

Lewis, N., and Reinhold, M. (1990). *Roman Civilization: The Republic and the Augustan Age*, Vol. 1. New York: Columbia University Press.

Lieberman, Saul (1955-1988). *Tosefta Kifushta: A Comprehensive Commentary on the Tosefta*. (Hebrew.) New York: Jewish Theological Seminary of America. Twelve Volumes.

Pliny (1952). *Natural History*, with an English translation by H. Rackman. Vol. IX, Books 33-35, Loeb Classical Library. Cambridge: Harvard University Press.

Radutsky, Elena (1993). The Education of Deaf People in Italy. In John Van Cleve, ed., *Deaf History Unveiled: Interpretations from the New Scholarship*. Washington, DC: Gallaudet University Press.

Safrai, Schmuel (Editor) (1987). *The Literature of the Sages: Oral Torah, Halakah, Mishna*, Tosefta, Talmud, External Tractates. Philadelphia: Fortress Press.

Saunders, Trevor J. (Tr.) (1981). *Aristotle: The Politics*. New York: Penguin books.

Shiffman, Lawrence H. (1991). *From Text to Tradition: A History of Second Temple Rabbinic Judaism*. Hoboken: Ktav Publishing House, Inc.

Shuchatowitz, Mordechai (undated). *Halacha Concerning Jewish Deaf and Hard of Hearing*. A publication of "Our Way" (a division of the Orthodox Union), 45 W. 36th Street, NY, NY 10018.

Strack, Hermann L., and Gunther Stemberger. (1996). *Introduction to the Talmud and Midrash*. Second Printing. Tr. M. Bockmuehl. Minneapolis: Fortress Press.

Winzer, Margaret A. (1997). Disability and Society Before the Eighteenth Century: Dread and Despair. In L. J. Davis, *The Disability Studies Reader*. New York: Routledge.

Wright, David (1969). *Deafness*. New York: Stein and Day Publishers.

doi: 10.1300/J095v10n03_07

Judaism, Theology and the Human Rights of People with Disabilities

Melinda Jones, BA, LLB

SUMMARY. How we understand Jewish attitudes to disability will depend on whether, like the reform movement, we take the torah to be the only relevant text, or whether our understanding of Judaism incorporates the "oral law," the Talmud. The belief that all human beings were created in the image of God presupposes an acceptance that each life is of

Melinda Jones is Research Associate, Faculty of Law at Monash University, Melbourne, Victoria, and Research Director of the B'nai B'rith Anti-Defamation Commission. She has written extensively on the subject of human rights, and is currently editing a book, *Critical Perspectives on Human Rights and Disability Law*, to be published by Kluwer in 2006. She is a Traditional Orthodox Jew, whose five children, including one with Cohen's Syndrome and an intellectual disability, have inspired her work. She has been actively involved in and for the Australian Jewish community, working to combat anti-Semitism and to promote the rights of people with disabilities.

[Haworth co-indexing entry note]: "Judaism, Theology and the Human Rights of People with Disabilities." Jones, Melinda. Co-published simultaneously in *Journal of Religion, Disability & Health* (The Haworth Pastoral Press, an imprint of The Haworth Press, Inc.) Vol. 10, No. 3/4, 2006, pp. 101-145; and: *Jewish Perspectives on Theology and the Human Experience of Disability* (ed: Rabbi Judith Z. Abrams, and William C. Gaventa) The Haworth Pastoral Press, an imprint of The Haworth Press, Inc., 2006, pp. 101-145. Single or multiple copies of this article are available for a fee from The Haworth Document Delivery Service [1-800-HAWORTH, 9:00 a.m. - 5:00 p.m. (EST). E-mail address: docdelivery@haworthpress.com].

inherent value to the creator despite apparent imperfections. The requirement to heal the world through deeds of loving kindness is incumbent on each and every Jew independent of disability and it is the responsibility of communities to remove any barriers there are to observance. Essentially, Judaism teaches us that one must treat others as they themselves would wish to be treated, and this extends equally to those who have disabilities. doi:10.1300/J095v10n03_08 *[Article copies available for a fee from The Haworth Document Delivery Service: 1-800-HAWORTH. E-mail address: <docdelivery@haworthpress.com> Website: <http://www.Haworth Press.com>* © *2006 by The Haworth Press, Inc. All rights reserved.]*

KEYWORDS. Human rights, Judaism, Halacha, equality, disability, inclusion, dignity

Theology involves "thinking" or "talking about" God, and invites questions about the existence of God, the nature of God, the relationship between God and humanity, and the relationship between God and religious practice. Theology leads to consideration of the meaning of life and death, and of human suffering, and encourages speculation about the possibility and significance of an afterlife. Evidence to support theological claims is to be found in the sacred texts of the tradition and in the folklore, stories and myths developed throughout the generations of communities of believers.

It is generally assumed that theological questions, debates and considerations are what makes a religion. While God is at the heart of Judaism and is present in all aspects of thinking and living, theological questions are almost tangential to the Jewish religious tradition. The vast majority of books on Judaism focus on questions other than theological ones. Judaism is primarily concerned with human behaviour and the question of what we need to do to become close to God. To establish this we are implored to study Torah, and to follow Jewish law.

> Despite the formidable intellectual energies Jews have devoted throughout the centuries to interpreting the will of God, they rarely wrote systematic theologies. They prayed to God and argued with Him, but they did not try to fit Him into the finite categories of human thought.[1]

This paper seeks to answer a number of specific questions about Jewish theology in relation to disability. First, what does Jewish theology tell us about people with disabilities, and more importantly, how does Jewish theology support or undermine the human rights of people with disabilities. Secondly, to what extent can Jewish thought provide a worldview that offers solace and hope to people with disabilities in the real world, and how does Jewish theology require society to respond to disability issues. Thirdly, I consider the questions of whether Jewish theology is consistent with the newly developed human rights framework for people with disabilities. Finally, I am concerned to establish whether the ideological imperative of an inclusive society in which diversity is celebrated and in which people with disabilities are treated with equality, concern and respect is consistent with Jewish theology. These considerations will provide insight into the place of people with disabilities in the Jewish world.

It is often argued that it is wrong to speak of Judaism as if it comprises one idea, ideology or theology just as it is wrong to assume that there is one Christian theology. Judaism, it is argued, is more accurately a reference to "Judaisms" which entail a range of theological understandings around the core ideas of the revelation at Mount Sinai, the belief in one and only one God, and the notion of chosen-ness. This view certainly provides a means of including within a discussion of Jewish theology the very different ideologies which emerge from Reform or Progressive Judaism, Conservative and Reconstructionist Judaism and mainstream or Orthodox Judaism. It gives equal status to the different Jewish denominations, and allows for there to be Jewish truths rather than a Jewish Truth.[2] It legitimizes the practices of all Jewish religious groups and organizations, and empowers those who believe themselves to be outsiders from mainstream Judaism.

The Chief Rabbi of Britain and the Commonwealth, Jonathon Sacks, takes a quite different view, however. He argues that, while there can be and is pluralism to be found in Jewish social life and practice, there is only one Judaism.[3] The plurality among Jews is certainly evident: there are Jews who consider themselves part of a race or culture and consider Judaism as religion as irrelevant; there are Jews who are completely assimilated, and others who believe the only relevance of Judaism is the identity of birth; there are Jews who are heterosexual and others who are homosexual; there are Jews who are committed to the empowerment of women and others who believe firmly in patriarchy; there are Jews who pray, perform Jewish rituals, and live their lives around structured religion; and there are Jews who believe that ethical conduct is the totality of Judaism. There are different expressions and interpretations of the obligations of Judaism and different lifestyles associated with this. There are Jews who consider that they live Jewish destiny to the full by living in Israel and have Zionism (Jewish nationalism) as their fundamental understanding of Judaism. There are others, living scattered into small communities across the entire world, speaking diverse languages and sharing the diverse majority cultural experiences of the societies in which they live. The plurality of Jewish experience is an uncontroversial fact and the diversity of cultural and social practices so great that Emanuel Kant and Hegel considered that Judaism is not a religion at all.[4] But for Chief Rabbi Sacks, there is only one legitimate version of Judaism. Those belonging to religious organizations which are non-Orthodox or non-mainstream may be very good people and very good Jews. They are, however, simply mistaken, confused or ignorant about the requirements of Jewish law.

Adopting the first perspective on Judaism complicates the task of understanding Jewish theology and understanding the relationship between Jewish theology, human rights and disability. Adopting the latter simplifies the task. While I am personally drawn to Chief Rabbi Sacks' argument, my political purpose suggests the acceptance of the Judaisms' perspective. My conclusion that Jewish theology supports a human rights account of people with disabilities, and that Judaism can therefore be brought in to bear on the secular discussions about the means of empowering people with disabilities, would be considerably weakened if it were to make sense only within the framework of Orthodox/mainstream/traditional Judaism. As such, I will set aside this debate, and continue my discussion of Jewish theology including alternative perspectives as variations on a theme, wherever they appear to be pertinent.

As a human rights scholar and disability activist, there are three reasons for examining Judaism and Jewish theology. The first is that a human rights model of disability takes all social and political institutions–including religion–to be potential sites of discrimination against people with disabilities. The discrimination may be subtle and not immediately apparent, as it may take the form of structural or ideological barriers to the full inclusion of people with disabilities. It therefore becomes incumbent on disability researchers to examine and disclose barriers operating within institutions, in this case within the purview of Jewish theology. Any aspects of Judaism which operate to prevent the participation of people with disabilities, on this account, require reanalysis and rectification.

The second reason for interrogating Judaism and Jewish theology is that, where it is found to be consistent with the human rights approach, it can provide an additional foundation for the ethical arguments surrounding human rights. While "rights" are based on exclusionary liberal constructions of the state, "human rights" attempt to transcend particular political ideologies and circumstances and to be universal and indivisible. My own interpretation of human rights is based on the inherent moral equivalence of all people, the correlative obligation to treat all people with equality, dignity and respect, and the aspiration for an inclusive society in which diversity is celebrated and individual difference valued. These ethical principles underlie human rights law, but currently have relatively weak articulation. If support for this ethical schema can be found in Jewish theology, the validity of my approach will be greater.

The third reason for my preliminary investigation of Jewish theology in terms of the human rights of people with disabilities is that it is hoped that this will spur other scholars to similarly challenge other religious systems and beliefs. Given that Judaism is very much a minority religion, and the Jewish people are few in number, whatever success my argument may have in bringing about social change for people with disabilities is necessarily limited. This essay represents a preliminary excursion into Jewish theology. Significantly more work needs to be done if there is to be any possibility of achieving and maintaining an inclusive society. It is hoped that this preliminary investigation of these questions will lead to further scholarship about Judaism and disability and to comparative analysis in other religious traditions.

Before I turn to my analysis of Jewish theology, it is necessary to clarify the inclusive principles of human rights and to explain the perspective on disability presented by a human rights model of disability.

HUMAN RIGHTS AND THE HUMAN RIGHTS OF PEOPLE WITH DISABILITIES

Recognition of the human rights of people with disabilities has been slow in coming. While the impetus for the modern movement of human rights was the atrocities of WWII, the impact of Nazi policies of eugenics as it related to people with disabilities has rarely played centre stage. The attempted genocide of the Jewish people in the Nazi Holocaust affronted the sensibilities of civilized democrats, despite the long history of antisemitism in which they were implicated. However, the abuse of people with disabilities during WWII was consistent with the eugenic philosophies of social Darwinists, health professionals and lawyers throughout the Western world. High profile, well-respected scholars and public figures joined Eugenic and Hygiene Societies which supported the wholesale sterilization of people with disabilities. This was such an acceptable position that liberal US Supreme Court Judge, Oliver Wendell Holmes did not hesitate in saying, in support of the medical violation of a young woman, "that three generations of imbeciles were enough."[5] Those people unfortunate enough to live with disabilities were tragedies, objects of pity; their lives were considered to be not worth living and their very existence provoked fear and disgust. People with disabilities were so marginalized that they rarely made it on to the political or social agenda. They were, truly, out of sight and out of mind.

The current international movement towards a Convention on the Rights of People with Disabilities is indicative of the extent to which the position of people with disabilities has changed over the last 30 years. The struggle for a clear legal articulation of the human rights of people with disabilities may take many years. But ultimately the success of law in achieving human rights is dependent on the extent to which the broader community truly accepts that, at a deep ethical and ideological level, people with disabilities are not aberrant but simply different and are not "objects" or means to an end, but are subjectively equal to those without disabilities. The idea of the moral equivalence of all people has strong philosophical roots. However, the extension of the idea of true equality to all people, at all places and at all times, has been hindered by assumptions about the centrality of "rationality," 'autonomy' and "self-determination." As characteristics of rights-bearers, women, children, people with disabilities and people from "primitive" societies were deemed outside the realm of rights which guaranteed social participation and social equality. In this way, notions of liberal rights operated as exclusionary categories of social action, and instead of promoting the rights of all people to be treated with equal concern and respect, operated to empower some while arbitrarily disempowering others. Before people with disabilities can possibly gain both the recognition and the benefits of equality, it is therefore necessary to replace liberal "rights-talk" with a democratic notion of human rights.

The central feature of a principled human rights approach is the desire for an inclusive society which celebrates diversity and dignifies difference, and in which all people are treated with dignity and respect. Human rights are universal and indivisible constructs, which insist on the inherent moral equivalence of all people. As such, the only laws and social actions which are respectful of the inherent dignity of all people are the only legitimate ones. This requires analysis of social arrangements and relationships to ensure that hidden barriers to equality are disclosed and disbanded. The responsibilities and duties that go with human rights belong not only to the state but also to all whose human rights are unproblematically protected. I have characterized my approach to human rights as a "MEDDICAL Model" of human rights. M and E represent moral equivalence; DD is for dignity in difference; I is for inclusion (and the objection to segregation); C is for the consciousness of how laws and rules operate at a systemic as well as overt level; A is Access or Accommodation–both required to ensure basic equality; and L could be for law, but is actually for learning, which can never cease because human rights require vigilance.

The application of principles of human rights to people with disabilities is complex. This is because of the range of personal experiences of disability, which is differentially affected by the range of pathological causes of disability. There is a wide variety of disabilities, from physical to sensory, to visual, to auditory, to intellectual or psychiatric disabilities. What is disabling about the "condition" will vary from person to person and from place to place. What is needed to be done is greatly affected by whether one lives in a developed or developing country or under a democratic or non-democratic political regime. In either case, a human rights approach challenges us to ensure that people with disabilities are equal members of society, and this is not possible unless equality is accepted as uncontroversial. For people with disabilities this will mean a rejection of the medical model of disability, which considered people with disabilities as "cases"–with individual pathology–in need of medical treatment and rehabilitation before being fit to enter (or reenter) society. This attitude to disability has ensured that disability was privatized and considered to be an individual or family problem, not a problem of the community as a whole. Yet it is now clear that, beyond the disempowerment of having a disability, the exclusion of people with disabilities is as much a social as a corporeal construction. The development of the social model of disability has led to an understanding of the way in which social structures, institutions and social values conspire to disenfranchise people with disabilities. The social model of disability discloses the hidden barriers which prevent the full inclusion of people with disabilities into the society at large. These barriers include accessible buildings, accessible information, and an accessible complaints-system. Further, barriers to inclusion operate at almost every level, every organization and every social institution operating in Western societies, and this includes within religion.

The task of those working to ensure that the human rights of people with disabilities are respected is to locate and deconstruct the barriers to inclusion. Religion is a site of oppression for people with disabilities, as people with disabilities are often excluded from religious communities or treated as "charity cases"–people on whom good works can be practiced. As objects of professional curiosity, people with disabilities were unable to own their subjective reality or to have this reality validated by the respect of the broader community. Without dismissing the significance of the personal embodied experience of disability, and the ongoing support needs of many people with disabilities, a different attitude and some relatively minor lateral thinking can completely change a person's experience of the world. If we begin with the assumption of the moral equivalence of all people, and the commitment of treating all people in a dignified, respectful manner, we can relatively easily take the next step of developing creative strategies to ensure inclusion. Providing for the human rights of people with disabilities is not just a matter of removing legal impediments or of changing overtly disablist policies–although these strategies are valuable in themselves. If this were all that is required we could simply draw on the experience of racism and sexism. However, while rectification of historic disadvantage equalizes opportunity by altering the starting line, it does not ensure that the race itself is fair. If some people walk, others run, and others are required to jump hurdles, should the different experience of the course be taken into account when assessing the comparative end-points? Any ordinary task can be considerably more difficult for some people to perform than others. Is this just the luck of the draw? No matter the cause of the difference, where a person is excluded, or effectively excluded, from any life activity because of a disability, any accommodation or adjustments to the environment which allow inclusion must be considered. To do otherwise is to show less respect for people with disabilities than one would for any other person.

HUMAN RIGHTS AND JEWISH THEOLOGY

The revelation at Mt Sinai, when God summoned the entire Jewish nation to receive the Torah, is the key identifying feature of Judaism. It is at this point that Jews become a nation, by accepting the obligations of being God's chosen people and by adopting a distinct code of law and practice which differentiated Jews from other monotheistic religions. The earlier commitment of Abraham to serve one incorporeal God distinguished our Jewish ancestors from the idolatrous peoples amongst whom they lived. But it is the experience of the Jewish people at Mt Sinai that forged Jewish identity, and which provides the fundamental underpinnings of Jewish existence. Gillman comments that

> Revelation is what brings God into relationship with a community of human beings. Without God's revelation . . . God would be irrelevant to the human enterprise, and Judaism would be purely a matter of peoplehood and culture alone.[6]

It is through an understanding of the Revelation at Mt Sinai that we gain an insight into the nature and existence of God. Of particular significance is the covenantal relationship between man and God established at Mt Sinai. Every Jewish soul was said to be present at Mt Sinai, so that the future generations took part in the commitment of the people to accept God and God's law. So central is the experience of the Exodus from Egypt, that every year at Pesach we are reminded that we need to recall or remember our personal presence in Egypt and the experience of being strangers in the land and of being rescued from oppression. God did not speak just to Moses. He spoke to the whole of Israel–to the weak and strong, the poor and the rich, the educated and the uneducated. After hearing the Ten Commandments, the people pleaded with Moses to ascend Mt Sinai and receive the Torah, as God's voice and presence made them afraid. However, God had revealed Himself to all the people, so there was no reason for belief to require a leader or medium.

From the outset, the relationship between man and God has been multidimensional. Moses ascended Mt Sinai to receive the Torah and returned to the celebration of a graven image–the Golden Calf. God approved of Moses' decision to smash the Tablets of Stone, on which He had written the Ten Commandments with His own finger, lest it, too, become an object of worship.[7] Moses returned to the mountain top and had to plead with God, who was inclined to wipe out the Jewish people. Moses learnt the prayer of repentance–the one that is still part of the daily service and a major feature of the Yom Kippur prayers. The Hebrew word for repentance is *Teshuvah*, literally "return." Moses pleaded on behalf of himself and the Jewish people, saying that not only were they all sorry, but also that they were determined to return to the ways of the Torah.

On its own, this was not enough to appease God's anger. So Moses argued with God, and told Him that destroying the Jewish people in the desert would make other nations disdain Him. What sort of God is it that would lead a people out of slavery only to have them die in the wilderness, he asked. God accepted the wisdom of Moses' words, but was still not convinced that genocide was inappropriate. Moses then took another tack, one typical of Jewish prophets and one that provides insight into the nature of the Jewish God. He reminded God that he had made a commitment, entered a Covenant with Abraham, Isaac and Jacob, to which God, for all His power, was bound. He had promised that He would make Israel a great nation, and God accepted that He must keep His word. This involvement with God–both the close, personal relationship between Him and the Jewish people, and His distant unprecedented Greatness–was the pattern of the relationship between man and God over the following 3,000 years.

It is the interpretation of what happened at Mt Sinai–the very nature of the Revelation–which is the basis of the division between Reform and Orthodox Jewry. Mainstream Judaism holds that the whole of the Torah was revealed to Moses at Mt Sinai. This includes both the Written Law and the Oral Law. While not recorded simultaneously with the Revelation, the Written Law or *Tanach* includes the Ten Commandments written on the Tablets of Stone, the Five Books of Moses, in Hebrew the *Chumash*, and a number of books which record events and guidance offered by various prophets, judges, kings and teachers–the Books of Prophets (*Nevi'im*) and Writings (*Ketuvim*). The Oral Law consists of teaching, interpretations and explanations of the Written Law as well as some supplementary material. This law was taught to Joshua, the elders and the rest of the people gradually over the years, passed on by word of mouth. This was a means of ensuring that it was understood by all of Israel who, living by the word of the Torah, were obliged to study and learn it. Only when many teachers and scholars were killed or imprisoned during the period of Roman rule, and then the people dispersed on the destruction of the 2nd Temple, was there fear that the Oral Law could be lost and a decision made to commit it to writing. Two parallel texts emerged over a number of generations–one from Jerusalem, the other from Babylon. Known as *Talmud*, the texts each contained the six orders of the *Mishna*, compiled by Rabbi Yehuda Ha Nasi at the end of the 2nd Century of the Common Era, and explanations and commentaries on the *Mishna* collected by successive generations of rabbis, referred to as *Gemara*. The *Jerusalem Talmud* was compiled by Rabbi Yochanan in Israel in the 4th century CE, and the *Babylonian*

Talmud by Ravina and Rav Ashi in the late 6th century. As Revealed Law, the whole of the Torah is authoritative and provides binding law for the governance of the whole Jewish people.[8]

This perspective on Revelation and the Torah, however, is rejected by Reform Judaism, which only accepts the authority of the Written Law. Referring to the Orthodox view as one of "Dual Torah," Reform Judaism considers the Oral Law to simply be a perspective on the Torah posited at one time, or over one period, and that the interpretation by the Rabbis is no more legitimate or authoritative than the opinions of Jewish scholars, philosophers or religious leaders at any other time. The difference between the two interpretations of the Revelation has dramatic consequences, for the different understandings of Revelation lead to quite different views about almost every aspect of Judaism and to different answers to almost every theological question.

One pertinent example of the significance of the view of Revelation relates to the perspective of Judaism on disability. Judith Abrams, a Reform Rabbi whose PhD thesis formed the basis of her important book, *Judaism and Disability*, argues that the Jewish position on disability is quite unacceptable today.[9] Because she draws her information on the Jewish attitude to disability solely from the Written Law, she focuses on rules about purity and Temple practices. She concludes that Jewish law is discriminatory because it supports an ideology of the "abnormality" "impurity" and "outsider status" of people with disabilities. She responds to her findings by arguing that Judaism needs to be updated and rewritten to include people with disabilities. On the other hand, because my own preliminary analysis of Jewish law is informed by Orthodox Judaism, I have come to the opposite conclusion about the Jewish conceptualisation of disability. Drawing on Rabbinical sources–the Oral Law–as well as on the Written Law of the Torah, I have argued that Jewish law is not culpable in the unjust treatment of people with disabilities. Rather, it is Jewish practice and the social action of Jews and Jewish communities which are at fault in the exclusion or abuse of the rights of Jewish people with disabilities. My response is that it is not Jewish law that is in need of updating or change, but rather that Jews need to take Jewish law more seriously if there is to be any possibility of an inclusive society.[10] Abrams looks at technical rules relating to worship; I look to the ethical code of conduct specified by Jewish law. Abrams finds fixed, inflexible characterisations of people with disabilities and beliefs about disability; I find a system supportive of vulnerable people and which seeks to empower the disempowered.

It is important to understand that my concern here is with Jewish thinking and Jewish theology rather than with Jewish practice. For the purpose of this essay it is irrelevant whether all or any Jews act consistently with the conclusions drawn (although one would very much hope that this would be the case). I am not concerned to present case studies of the experience of Jewish people with disabilities, nor to consider whether one strand of Judaism is better or worse at including people with disabilities in their community. Recognizing that most people with disabilities experience inequality and human rights abuses on a daily basis, no existing religious or other institution satisfactorily protects the human rights of people with disabilities. I believe that the only way of achieving the change required for people with disabilities to have a more "normal" life is for the beliefs and attitudes about disability and about people with disabilities to be interrogated, and for existing assumptions to be transformed into new common sense assumptions that inclusion and moral equivalence are "right" and anything undermining these principles is "wrong." If my interpretation of Jewish theology is correct, it is consistent with the world view I am proposing, so translating theology into action becomes central to the possibility of justice for people with disabilities.

If, on the other hand, Jewish theology is inconsistent with these principles, my hope would be that there would be a re-examination of Jewish law, Halacha, to adjust it to modern values. The ability of Halacha to adapt and to provide solutions for new types of issues arising in societies very different from where it first held sway is, possibly, its greatest achievement. Halacha literally means "the way." It comprises laws concerning man's relationship with God, and man's relationship with man. The commands directed at people regarding the treatment of their fellows are inherent aspects of man's relationship with God. There are significant problems, from a mainstream or Orthodox perspective on Judaism, with changing Halacha, although change is not impossible.[11] Other Judaisms take a more flexible approach. Unless it transpires that there is a problem with existing law, this is not a hurdle I need to jump at this point.

GOD–HIS NATURE AND ATTRIBUTES

The Jewish God is both transcendent and immanent. This is not as paradoxical as it may seem. God is infinite, absolute, limitless, universal, incorporeal, indivisible and ultimately, according to Maimonides, unknowable.[12] He is the Creator of the Universe. On the other hand,

God is to be found everywhere, close to us; within reach should we seek to find Him. God is just and merciful, generous, compassionate and demanding. He is pleased or displeased with human behavior, and "rests" on the Shabbat. He clothes the naked and buries the dead. He brings food to the hungry and visits the sick. He is emotional–cries, laughs, smiles, scowls, gets angry and feels pity. He is sometimes a parent–loving and nurturing, closely involved with every move we make; critical of our actions, giving strict guidance to our activities. At other times, God as parent will show restraint in the face of our maturity to allow us room to make our own mistakes. He is neither male nor female, the parenting He provides is often said to comprise both the ideals of motherly and fatherly love. The gendered references to God as "He" are a matter of convention, and references to "our Father, our King" and to "Lord" and "Master" are indicative of the poverty of language to encapsulate an idea beyond human imagining.

The names used for God are chiefly taken from His ethical attributes: "The world's Righteous One," "The Merciful One," and most frequently "The Holy One, blessed be He." God calls Himself "I am who I am," the Source of all existence, above all things, independent of all conditions, and without any physical quality.[13] We are told that God is the "God of gods" because "He is exalted above any conception of Him of which man is capable."[14] Nontheless, God is not considered to be an abstract idea. He is a dynamically powerful living God, who continues the act of creation throughout the existence of time. He is anything but an absentee landlord–a creator who set the world in motion, then left it to run itself. His presence is essential for the ongoing functioning of the world. Man and morality could not exist without God. "He constantly does things which are totally 'impossible' and defy definition."[15]

The Jewish commitment to God involves an uncompromising monotheism.[16] God is One, Unique, Indefinable and Indivisible. Beyond this point, Judaism leaves considerable freedom in the explanations of God. However inadequate a definition of God may be, all attempts to provide an understanding of the nature of God are legitimate. Because God is inherently beyond the confines of the human mind and beyond our imagination, all anthropomorphic references in the Bible, whether to God's arm, face, back, hand or finger, are necessarily metaphorical. To think otherwise would be to suggest God is corporeal, and this reaches very close to idolatry.[17] Steinhaltz comments that: "The understanding of God as 'the completeness of everything' is quite simple, and it is not an anthropomorphic picture of God."[18]

BELIEF IN GOD

> Since God is altogether beyond us, there is no way to prove Him, because if we could, He would be confined to the limits of our minds! This would be a contradiction in terms! . . . If it were proven beyond doubt that God exists, then much of humanity's freedom of choice would be restricted. Man would be forced to follow God's instructions and one would have no choice but to follow the moral code (free will re good and evil no longer relevant).[19]

Belief in God is taken for granted by all but a small minority of Jewish thinkers.[20] Because we were all present at Mt Sinai, we have experienced God, so have direct knowledge of His existence. Discussion of God proceeds on the basis that there is one and only one God, and within Judaism this is axiomatic. One Talmudic discussion of God compares God to the sun, in order to explain how much greater is God than any aspect of the universe. Rabbi Joshua ben Hananiah explains to a Caesar that he cannot see God, but Caesar is insistent. So Rabbi Joshua instructed that he look directly at the sun. When Caesar objects that he cannot, Rabbi Joshua responds: "If you say of the sun, which is only one of the servitors standing before the Holy One, blessed be He, 'I cannot look directly at it', how much less could you look at the Presence (Shekhenah) itself?"[21]

Questioning is the hallmark of Jewish thinking. Emanuel Rackman commented that "Judaism encourages doubt even as it enjoins faith and commitment. A Jew dares not live with absolute certainty, because certainty is the hallmark of the fanatic and Judaism abhors fanaticism, [and] because doubt is good for the human soul, its humility . . . "[22] Even Abraham and Moses questioned God, and challenged His ability to do the impossible. When God told Abraham and Sarah (who were 99 & 89 years old respectively) that they were to have a child, they doubted His word. Abraham suggested a line from Ishmael would be more realistic, but God simply responded: "Is anything too hard for the Eternal?"[23] Similarly, when God promised Moses that He would provide meat for the Children of Israel while they wandered in the desert, Moses was not convinced that this was possible–even after witnessing the Plagues in Egypt and the miracle of the parting of the Red Sea. God's response was: "And the Eternal said, is the Eternal's hand short?"[24] When God does not answer our prayers, for the possible or impossible, it is not that God is unable to respond. It is rather that, for a reason which we may not be able to fathom, God has chosen His course of action.

God created the Universe with a purpose, and Judaism believes that everything in the world is also a part of that purpose. The story is told of a Chassidic Rabbi whose student asked the purpose of heresy. His response was that "when you confront another who is in need, you should imagine that there is no God to help, but that you alone can meet the man's needs."[25] In a similar vein, you cannot discard your obligation to act justly towards a needy person because of a belief that they will be rewarded in the world to come. God requires that we act now to relieve distress or oppression.[26] For people with disabilities this should provide some hope, as it means that all Jews have an obligation to respond to the injustice around them.

Judaism considers that God is less about power than about relationships. While God can be found in nature and in man, He is not equivalent to either nature or man. God does not wish to remain hidden from humanity, but it is in our court to find Him. Yet Judaism does not require the "faith" of adherents, in the normal meaning of the term; rather, the Hebrew word *Emunah* means faithfulness or loyalty to God, rather than "faith." Over a thousand years ago, Rabbi Saadia Gaon wrote that "[f]aith was never regarded by Judaism as a consecrated act on which salvation depends; it is considered of value only insofar as it leads to right action."[27] According to the Talmud, God Himself declared "Better that they [the Jews] abandon Me, but follow My laws";[28] the Rabbis added that whereas a man or woman may begin to practice Judaism for reasons unrelated to God, such as seeing the rule as rational or as consistent with the person's ethical commitments, he or she will eventually do so because of God.[29]

We are to be faithful to God, and to place our trust in His hands. When Abraham was commanded to leave his home in Ur, he was not told the destination. On the faith that God would follow through, Abraham left everything familiar to him and went to a place which "I shall show you."[30] Abraham's greatness was his preparedness to undertake the journey, to walk with God. For us, the journey into the unknown, towards God, is a means of finding ourselves. God is within us; He is available to all who seek Him.

HUMANITY–THE WORTH OF THE INDIVIDUAL

[God] brought the universe into being as a parent conceives a child, acting not blindly but out of love. We are not insignificant, nor are we alone. We are here because someone willed us into being, who wanted us to be, who knows our innermost thoughts, who values us in our uniqueness, whose breath we breathe and in whose arms we rest; someone in and through whom we are connected to all that is.[31]

This is true, independent of any characteristics we may have. What is true for any of us is equally true for a person with a disability. Jewish theology holds that we are all created by God and can all trace our heritage to Adam. Man was made from the dust and the breath of God. This results in each of us having a soul, in Hebrew *Neshama*, a spark of the Divine. Beyond this link with God, however, is another fundamental feature of Man. "God made man in His own image; in the image of God He created him; male and female He created them."[32] The use of the plural and the repetition is to emphasize that we are all, without distinction, made in God's image. At the time of the Bible and throughout history, the idea that all people–not just Kings or Princes or the elite–were all made in God's image, was a radical idea.[33] Today we pay lip service to guarantees of rights or assumptions of equality. The 20th century saw atrocity after atrocity: facism, totalitarianism and the Cult of Personality degraded man by making him bow down to the brute exercise of power. Judaism elevated man by declaring him to be the culmination of creation, God's agent on earth, made in God's image.

Different interpretations of the meaning of being made in God's image include: a distinction between animals and humanity; the possibility of intellectual perception; the ability to reason; the experience of emotions; the ability to create; the existence of moral character, by which we can know good from evil. Given how different we are from each other–variety being on a range of axis: language, culture, gender, race, ability, appearance, intelligence/IQ, material possessions, socioeconomic position, age, etc.–the fact that we are all created in God's image both unifies us and is evidence that God loves diversity. No feature or characteristic makes us less or more important; we are each of fundamental importance independent of social judgment. "Beloved is man who is created in God's image";[34] so who could be so presumptuous to say "my blood is redder than yours"?[35] Being made in God's image also requires that we are God-like in our actions. We must reflect God's characteristics, because it is our capacity to do justice, to be merciful and to keep our promises which distinguish us as humans.

The fact that God initially created Adam alone has been seen as further evidence of the importance of each and every individual. Just as there is one God, there was at first one man. Noone can claim that they have superior parentage, or that their father is greater than another's. No person is of greater value than another. None are more worthy or more significant than another. We are morally equivalent– different yet equal; the same yet distinct. The shape of our body and the sharpness of our minds are totally irrelevant. People with disabilities are equally valuable, equally important, equally entitled to share in the benefits of society. To the extent that it is possible to attribute human rights to anybody, they apply equally to all. In Judaism, then, we find support for the moral claim of people with disabilities to be considered as equal, valuable people totally independent of ANY aspect of their disability. Siegel makes a similar point: "if all humanity does have a common origin, it is obvious, then, that the disabled or handicapped are not derived from an alien source which is 'inferior,' since all have a common source."[36]

The principle of the fundamental value of human life is also said to be derived from Adam's singular creation. "Whoever destroys one life, it is as if he has destroyed an entire world. Whoever saves one life, it is as if he has saved an entire world."[37] Telushkin explains that, as a consequence, saving many lives at the expense of one life is not permitted; by definition many infinities cannot be worth more than one infinity.[38] The life-saving principle does not allow for any distinction to be made between people, as *all* life is infinite. This clearly applies to the able as well as the disabled.

Not only does Judaism hold that every person is of equal worth, it also considers that every moment of every life is of infinite value. This is not contingent on good health or an able body. Therefore Judaism rejects totally the notion that some lives are not worth living. This is not for us to judge. As our bodies belong to Hashem, we cannot damage them in any way.[39] The Biblical command: "you shall, therefore, keep my statutes and my ordinances, which if a man do he shall live by them"[40] has been interpreted by the Rabbis to mean "you shall live by them, not die by them."[41] When life is at stake, other laws must be set aside.[42] For Rabbi Heschel the life-saving principle is the mark of humanity: "So why should the life and dignity of an individual man be regarded as infinitely precious? . . . [because every] human being is a disclosure of the Divine."[43]

This principle is extremely important for people with disabilities. Deformed babies are no longer exposed as a matter of course, as they have been throughout history. However, the media constantly reinforces the association of disability with moral deformity (evil) which needs to be defeated by unblemished superheroes. Given the message that deviation from the norm is unacceptable, the reassurance that a disabled life is as precious and as entitled to exist as an able life is crucial. While eugenic programs designed to eradicate disability are no longer in vogue, the logic of the eugenics movement underpins the massive investment in the Human Genome Project. This poses a threat to people with disabilities before they are born and at any stage when it is decided that living a life with a disability is a waste of resources and is expendable as a life not worth living. From a Jewish perspective, these lives are as worthy as any other lives. As Abraham comments: "We have no yardstick by which to measure the worth and importance of a life, not even in terms of the person's knowledge of Torah and the fulfillment of Mitzvot. One must set aside the Shabbat laws even for a person who is old and sick, who may be socially unacceptable because of a repulsive external disease, who may be mentally retarded and incapable of performing any Mitzvot."[44]

The view that disabled lives are not worth living has a number of current manifestations. Dominant among these is the position that killing people with disabilities may be both morally and legally permissible. Acceptance of mercy killing and euthanasia are wipespread, justified by the view that no rational person could possibly want to live his or her life if marred by the existence of a disability and that, given the option, s/he would rather be dead. While a person may think that he/she would rather be dead than live in a particular state, this is rarely the position that person adopts on reaching that state.[45] The question of whether the person consented to die, and that the murderers were simply assisting suicide, is certainly not provable once the person is dead. However, where euthanasia is legal, as it is in the Australian Northern Territory, a cloud hangs over all people with disabilities. Whenever a decision is made that the life in question is not worth living (and, given the attitude of many to people with disabilities, this could often be assumed to be the case), the person could and possibly should be "assisted" to end his or her life.[46] The response of Judaism to mercy killings, euthanasia, assisted-suicide and assumptions that there could be any life that is not worth living, is clear. All life is of the utmost value,[47] and this is so whether or not disability is involved. Judaism recognizes that all people are of equal, infinite and ultimate value, even though people vary considerably in ability, personality, shape and size. Life is a gift, to be treated with respect. Nothing could be more valuable, and noone is less valuable.[48]

MORALITY, SIN AND SUFFERING

[t]he very essence of the Torah acknowledges the possibility of human failure. Implementation of the Torah is built on the premise that man could fail. The commandments presuppose non-obedience! Sinai shows real people who are vulnerable and weak. And still, God is prepared to get involved.[49]

Judaism is not only a living religion but is also a religion for the living. While we are made in God's image, there is no person "so wholly righteous on earth that he will always do good and will never sin."[50] This is because we are afflicted or blessed with the *Yetzer Ha'ra* (the evil inclination) and the *Yetzer Ha'tov* (good inclination), and have potential both to make good choices and bad choices. Torah dictates all aspects of life: from toileting and bathing on waking; to the words we use and the thoughts we utter; from the way we treat those we know and the way we respond to strangers; from the way we see the world to the way we conceive our role in it; and from the moment we rise in the morning until the moment we take our rest at night. It is therefore impossible to get it right all the time.[51] However, "Halacha recognizes man's weaknesses and creates a way through which one is able to overcome his weaknesses within the boundaries of his ethical behavior."[52]

Human perfection is impossible and the idea tautological. By definition humans are in God's image, but are not and cannot be gods. We are all equal in imperfection and we all are required to strive towards godliness. The task of the Jew is to work to heal the world (*tikkun olam*) and to leave the world in a better state than when we entered it.[53] No one is exempt from this obligation and, while our abilities to perform some of the commandments may vary, the fact of being a person with disabilities is irrelevant to this duty. Whenever a bad deed is performed, it is said to tip the balance of the world towards evil; whenever a good deed is performed, it is said to tip the scale towards heaven.

The Hebrew word for sin is "Het" which literally means "to err." In sinning, one has made an error of judgment, made a mistake.[54] The assumption is that a person does not, generally, intentionally sin. While this is sometimes the case, the Jewish understanding of sin and response to sin is based on the fundamental preference of us all to do good. Judaism offers a solution to sin, other than suffering: the idea of *Teshuvah*, repentance, offers the possibility of an immediate release from sin. The word *teshuvah* literally means "return," and it is through *teshuvah* that one can return to a positive life. Just as there are laws governing the relationship between man and God and between man and man, sinful action can either be directed at God or at man. The process of Teshuvah for transgressions against God was outlined in the discussion of the Revelation, above. However, where the sin involved is a transgression of the proper relationship between man and man, then the solution is to be found between man and man, and asking God's forgiveness is of no consequence.[55] God does not resolve inter-personal issues of bad conduct. In the Jewish tradition, the forgiveness can only to be given by the one who is harmed by the sinful behavior. This is a pragmatic and worldly means of overcoming individual acts of evil–admitting one was wrong, saying sorry, feeling remorse, and committing to refrain from such behavior in the future. In the Book of Proverbs we are told that "[t]o do righteousness and justice is more acceptable to God than sacrifices"[56] Ironically, every sin provides its author with the opportunity to become a better person.

The idea of Satan as an evil power, equal and opposite to God, is a heretical idea. No other creative force can exist beside God. He made both the light *and* the darkness and created in humanity both the force for good and the option of evil, together with the faculty of free ethical choice. Humanity is not tarnished by the "original sin" of Adam's "fall" from the Garden of Eden. Given that "to err is to be human," Judaism considers that it would be irrational for God to condemn humans for sinning.[57] The major "punishment" of giving in to the evil inclination, is to lower the worth of the sinner in his or her own eyes as well as in the eyes of the community. Sinning, therefore, is really letting oneself down. Equally, performing good deeds is of psychological benefit to the actor. It is much easier to like oneself and to feel good about the world when one has controlled the temptation to speak ill of another, has visited a sick person, or made another person feel good about herself, than it is when one has compromised oneself by failing to perform a mitzvah. From a Jewish perspective, it is the choices we make and our responses to these impulses, particularly resisting the *yetzer hara,* which ultimately determines who we are.[58]

The concept of free will is fundamental to Judaism. If we were unable to make moral choices it would make no sense to talk of commandments, prohibitions, reward and punishment. We are commanded to exercise the faculty of choice in a meaningful way, and to take responsibility for our actions. God makes this clear: "I have set before you life and death, blessing and curse. Choose life so that you and your offspring may live."[59] Schroeder explains that the price of making bad decisions, big or small, is death, and that we should therefore take our ethical obligations very seriously.[60] "One should always stir up his good inclination against his evil inclination."[61] Jews are taught to regard themselves as stronger than sin, able to fight off all temptations. Curiously, Judaism assumes the greater the person, the greater the passion for sin. The solution, though, is not to become a recluse or an ascetic, but to take one's stand in the community. A person who overcomes the desire to break a law in the face of temptation is greater than the person who avoids having to make decisions. For example, it is no credit to eat only Kosher, when that is all that is available, but it is a good deed, a mitzvah, to refrain from eating pork when it is a commonplace part of the diet of the general population. Maimonides commented: "Free will is granted to every man. If he wants to accustom himself to righteousness and become righteous, he is free to do so; and if he wants to follow evil and become wicked, he is free to do so . . . "[62]

Judaism holds that good and evil are objective realities that transcend personal and national opinions; that there is a basis for morality that goes beyond the subjective ideals of individuals or society and insists that without God all morality is subjective: "morality ungrounded in God is indeed a house built upon sand, unable to stand up against the vagaries of impulse and the brutal pressures of power and self-interest."[63] Without God we would have no way of knowing right from wrong, and we would be unable to have any context into which we exercise our free will. However, where there is free will it is inevitable that bad things must happen and sometimes bad things will happen to good people. The story of Cain and Abel demonstrates this: "Cain murdered Abel. It was Abel whose sacrifice was accepted by God. If Abel was the good guy, why didn't God protect him? Two aspects of biblical religion arise from this: bad things happen, and God lets them happen."[64] Schroeder explains that an omnipotent Creator could easily stop the Cains before they acted, "but that would be inconsistent with free will. As long as choice is ours, the possibility for evil, often unintentionally inflicted, exists."[65]

Bad things that arbitrarily happen to good people should be compared with the randomness of the natural universe. Alongside the "normal" blue skies, rain, thunder and lightening, we recognize drought and flood and earthquakes as random parts of the scheme of nature. Schroeder argues that the experience of bad along with good is the price we pay for free will. Without some degree of randomness, all events and all choices in the universe would be totally predetermined by unyielding laws of nature, the physics and the chemistry of all reactions. We would be mere robots. Our every thought and action would be fixed by the immediately preceding chemistry of our bodies and the conditions of the environment. The future would be totally controlled by the past."[66]

On this account, the cause of disability is random. Disabilities acquired at birth are not Divine punishment for the sins of the parents. In fact, it is sometimes said that the birth of a child with disabilities is a form of respect for the parents chosen to carry out the task of nurturing the particular child. Disabilities acquired after birth are often a matter of being in the wrong place and the wrong time: industrial accidents, traffic injuries, falls on the football field, etc. These are not part of a Divine plan, but an inevitable consequence in living in an uncontrolled world. Jewish thinking consistently holds that disability is not a punishment for sin,[67] and that there is no moral deviance attached to being a person with a disability.[68] On the contrary, Judaism values "disabled lives" as much as any life, and people with disabilities are indispensable members of the community. The founder of the 18th Century Hassidic movement explained that the Jewish people are a living *Sefer Torah*, and *every living Jew* is one of its letters. As a Torah is *treiff* (unkosher) if it has even one letter rubbed out or incorrectly formed, this places an enormous burden on each individual to play her role in perfecting the world.[69] The reference to a letter which is "rubbed out or incorrectly formed" bears no relation to a person's ability or disability; rather, it refers to a person who fails to perform the *Mitzvot*–God's law. The Hassidic movement believes that when every Jew practices Judaism to the fullest, the *Mashiach* will come. Perfection of the world does not refer to human ideals of perfection, but to the ideal of humans who celebrate God's presence in all their lives. People with disabilities are needed, just as are the sick, the weak, the poor, or the vulnerable, for without their involvement in Judaism, we will never reach the goal of humanity.

The question of why bad things happen to good people is one that is not easily answered. The quintessential example of individual suffering is found in the Book of Job. Job loses everything–his family, his wealth, his health. One terrible thing after another happens to him, but he does not accept his friends' reasoning that he is being punished for his sins or the sins of his fathers. Job's faith remains unaltered, even though it is tested as one crisis follows another. At the end of the story Job is not rewarded and no explanation of his experience is offered to him. However, Job simply accepts that a mere human cannot expect to understand the reasoning of God who, despite Job's test, is known to be good and just.

The Holocaust did not separate good people from bad people, did not question whether the Jew was spiritual, religious, law-abiding or not.

Being a righteous Jew is no guarantee of the good life–at least in the sense of being protected from being afflicted with tragedy of one sort or another. However, being a righteous Jew has a different sort of reward. To the extent that the Jew is able to rejoice in the workings of God, and to appreciate and perhaps show wonder at His creations, the life of that Jew will be far richer than those who are too busy to celebrate the world around them. "It is for us to learn how to react to the bad as well as to the good even if we cannot understand the purpose of either."[70]

Harold Kushner, a rabbi whose son had a disability and a chronic degenerative disorder, argued that the wrong question is being asked by those who seek an answer to why they, personally, have bad things happen to them or to those who they love.[71] He argues that God is not involved in the life of individuals as directly as the question suggests. The effect of his argument, however, is that there are matters to which God's power cannot extend, and that in this respect God is limited. Schroeder responds that "Biblically there is no foundation for such an idea. Famines and holocausts do not occur because God is limited. The Bible itself informs us repeatedly that through *tsimtsum* [the contraction of the universe] and the occasional hiding of the divine presence, God allows them to happen as part of the divine scheme. What seems to be divine indifference lies not in some inherent limit to the Creator. Rather it is the foundation of our free will."[72] Further, it is man, not God, who is limited. Our failure to understand why bad things happen to good people is a result of our inherent inability to understand God.

THE ESSENCE OF JUDAISM

The Torah is to the soul of man what rain is to the soil; rain makes any seed put into the soil grow, producing nourishing as well as poisonous plants. The Torah also helps him who is striving for self-perfection, while it increases the impurity of heart of those that remain uncivilized.[73]

The Torah is the backbone of Judaism, and it is through study of the Torah that we learn what God requires of us and how to behave in an ethical manner.[74] We are told how to live our lives to the fullest and how to behave in virtually every situation. The Torah contains 613 commandments, all of which are important and all of which should be complied with to the best of the individual's ability.[75] The Torah also contains discussions and minority and majority opinions about what is meant by a particular rule and how one needs to act in order to fulfill the mitzvah (commandment). There are four categories of Jewish laws: reflexive laws; laws of ethics; laws of holiness; and national laws.[76] All categories of laws involve specific acts, some of which are ritualistic. However, performing a ritual is only a part of any law.

Reflexive laws are those which provide room for the individual to reflect on the world and on their place in it. The Hebrew word for prayer is l'hitpallel which means "to judge or examine oneself." The form of the verb is reflexive, suggesting that prayer is about the person engaged in prayer, and is designed to elevate the person. Prager and Telushkin go so far as to say that "God does not need our prayer, we do."[77] Prayers are very personal, although they take a fixed form. They extol the virtues of God and give praise to His majesty. Every person is able to pray, and while the prayers are written in Hebrew, Judaism accepts that God understands us, whatever language we speak. Of particular interest to people with disabilities is the importance of prayer in the context of illness.[78] Although people with disabilities are not necessarily unwell, and disability is usually disabling in the context of social action, not medical practice, my personal experience of disability has been frequent encounters with the medical profession, hospital stays and the daily reality of dysfunctional bodies requiring medical intervention. It is greatly uplifting when people recite Psalms on your behalf, in aid of recovery of illness or survival through surgery.

The categories of laws concerned with ethics are the most important for our purposes, as laws of ethics are concerned with the relationship between people. There are laws to do with the way we speak and the words we say; laws concerned with sexual conduct and sexuality; laws concerned with every imaginable aspect of business relations; laws concerned with hospitality; laws concerned with visiting the sick; laws to deal with justice and charity; laws relating to the treatment of the poor or oppressed; laws about burying the dead and comforting the mourner; and laws to do with marriage, divorce, family relationships and the way children are to behave towards their parents. There are also a number of ethical rules pertaining to the treatment and care of animals. These commandments are of particular importance for people with disabilities and the human rights of people with disabilities. For questions about the human rights of people with disabilities are essentially about the attitudes and values of those in the community without disability towards those with disabilities.

The laws of holiness are those laws designed to turn the mundane experiences of everyday life–such as eating, engaging in acts of sexual intimacy or noting the beauty in the world around us–into encounters with Hashem. Judaism does not consider that bodily experiences or pleasures are in any way sinful (although excess in all things is prohibited). Rather, we can be elevated from our animal selves by appreciating the world around us, by thinking about what we are doing rather than acting reflexively, and by communicating our joy of the world to God. This should lead to humility and optimism in the individual, who stops long enough to feel blessed by whatever they have. Judaism objects to the "fine fat lady who walks through the field in gloves, missing so much and so much." It is important to understand that holiness takes place through living in the world, and asceticism and reclusive behavior are not condoned. Further, the prophet Isaiah said: "The holy God is made holy through righteousness [not holiness]."[79]

National laws are religiously endorsed cultural events that mark Judaism as a community. These include the celebrations of religious festivals such as the Shabbat, Pesach and Purim. These are unimportant for our purposes, except to the extent that there is no basis on which the law applies differently from one person to the other.[80] All these laws are suspended when a person's life or health are at risk, and there are rulings about how to manage particular laws if one is ill or for some medical-type reason cannot adhere to the strictness of the law. There is enormous flexibility within the boundaries of the law, and no reason why anyone should be excluded from participation in any celebration. Of course, where the law involves attendance at a Shule or synagogue and the venue is inaccessible, the onus is on the community to make it possible for the person to be included in a manner that is both respectful and dignified. If this means redesigning or adapting a building to allow wheelchair access, for example, then the community, not the individual, is responsible to make adjustments to the best of its ability. A community which claims to include everyone, but makes particular abilities (such as the ability to walk up stairs) a condition of participation, or which treats some individuals with disrespect, is unacceptable in the eyes of God.

From the perspective of an ideal construction of orthodox or mainstream Judaism, all of these commandments are binding. No group is more important than the other, and there is a theological expectation that every act performed will consist of both *ma'aseh*, the deed or content, and *kavana*, the spirit or intention. However, the commandments include both positive and negative commandments, and while there can be no time at which a person can disobey a negative law, such as not to kill or not to steal, positive laws such as visiting the sick or providing hospitality are not required to be performed at every time of every day. Ideally, an orthodox Jew will be sufficiently preoccupied with these laws that noone can accuse him or her of neglecting the Torah. Telushkin makes the comments that if you were to "[a]sk any Jew–religiously observant or not–whether another Jew is religious, and the question is invariably answered by noting the person's observance of Jewish rituals, not of Jewish ethics. As if God regarded ethical observance as a voluntary, extra credit activity."[81]

There is a great deal of current, as well as historical, concern about the failure of many orthodox individuals to take the ethical laws of Judaism seriously. The Talmud asks: "if someone studies Bible and Mishna . . . but is dishonest in business and discourteous in his relations with people, what do people say about him? 'Woe unto him who studies the Torah . . . This man studied the Torah; look how corrupt his deeds, how ugly his ways' "[82] In a similar vein, Rabbi Lopes Cardozo comments that: "Orthodoxy potentially is picking and choosing between mizvot (the crime of Reform & Conservative) whenever it pleases when it decides the only commandments it takes seriously relate to ritual or Man-to-God commandments. Authentic Judaism requires as much if not more attention to ethical rules–man-to-man–which require exercise of freewill."[83]

Rabbi Salanter, founder of the Musar movement, illustrated the importance of complying with the ethical dictates of the Torah during the period when Tsar Nicholas I was forcing Jewish boys into the Russian army for 25-year terms. On visiting a small community, he chanced upon a widow sobbing bitterly. It transpired that she had been told that a second of her sons was to be conscripted into the Russian army, despite a communal agreement that no family would be required to send more than one child until every family had lost a child in this way. The son of a wealthy leader of the community was to have been drafted, but his father exercised his power and convinced the rest of the community that none of his children should be taken. In response, Rabbi Salanter attended the afternoon prayers and prevented man after man from leading the service by insisting that those who are not believers in God are forbidden to lead the prayers. When he was challenged, Rabbi Salanter is said to have responded that believers in God would not oppress widows or favor prominent people in a judgment, and that while they ignored these laws they were unfit to lead the service.

An alternative schema for classifying Halacha, distinguishes between *hukkim* and *mishpatim*. The former include the laws between man and God, and can be seen as laws of arbitrary Divine decree or laws which do not simply reflect the laws that we could come up with on our own. These include almost all of the ritual elements of Judaism–from observance of festivals, to laws seen as primarily symbolic, such as the wearing of a *tallit* or the fixing of a *mezuzah* on the door posts of our houses. The latter laws, *mishpatim*, comprise civil laws and laws of ethical conduct. It is said of the *mishpatim* that these are laws which humanity could have arrived at on its own without God's intervention. It is on this division of laws that Reform, Conservative and other alternative constructions of Judaism, depend. Neil Gillman comments: "Rituals, then, are practices that have no obvious interpersonal or ethical impact and no rational basis; they are binding simply because they are said to represent God's explicit will for us. Is it any wonder, then, that many of us have trouble making sense of these practices?"[84] In part because some practices are difficult and strange to a non-practicing Jew, Reform Judaism takes the theological position that *hukkim* are symbolic and binding only to the extent that they are of communal value.

From the perspective of people with disabilities, the question about Halacha, law and ritual is whether people with disabilities are included or excluded and whether there is any theological perspective that promotes the value of disabled lives and incorporates a view of the entitlement to be treated with dignity and respect. At this stage it is very clear that Judaism is available for people with disabilities, in the sense that there is no exclusion from either the obligations of the law or of the benefits of the law. Despite theological differences, there is agreement that the various attempts to reduce Judaism to its essence capture the important requirements of and for people with disabilities. This is because in almost every case the emphasis has been on ethical conduct. The most famous attempt to encapsulate Judaism in a single phrase is that of Hillel. The story is told of a person interested in converting to Judaism in the first century Before the Common Era. He approached the two leading sages of the age to summarize Judaism while standing on one foot. The first, Shammai, sent him away, but Hillel is said to have responded: "what is hateful to you, do not do to your neighbor. This is the whole Torah, the rest is commentary–now go and study."[85] By casting the Golden Rule in negative relief, Hillel simplifies the task of unpacking the meaning of the commandment, while retaining the requirement of studying Torah both for its own sake and in order to understand the true meaning of the principle.

In another famous discussion about the heart of Judaism, the Talmud records the words of Rabbi Akiva and Rabbi Ben Azzai. Taking the statement 'Ye shall love your neighbor as yourself' from the Book of Leviticus,[86] Rabbi Akiva said "[T]his is the major principle of the Torah." To this Rabbi Ben Azzai responded, " '[t]his is the book of generations of Man'[87]–this is a greater principle of the Torah."[88] Rabbi Ben Azzai was referring to the statement that man is made in God's image, which he considered to be even more fundamental to the practice of Judaism than the Golden Rule. If we recall that being made in God's image involves the inherent value and dignity of every person, and that this moral equivalence of people is to be reflected in every human action or endeavor, we can conclude that the full range of readings of Jewish theology support the human rights of people with disabilities.

COMING CLOSE TO GOD

> They found God in the mystery and majesty of the personal. Hearing God reach out to man, they began to understand the significance of human beings reaching out to one another. They began, haltingly at first, to realize that God is not about power but relationship; that religion is not about control but about freedom; that God is found less in nature than in human society, in the structures we make to honor His presence by honoring His image in other human beings. Biblical faith is about the dignity of the personal, and it can never be obsolete.[89]

The Torah itself presents us with the problem of how it is possible to come close to God, given that we know that no man can see God and live. The usual way of become close to God is through prayer and worship or by acting in a spiritual manner. However, this is not the Jewish means of coming close to God. The Talmudic discussion of the question focuses on the commandment: "You shall follow after the Lord your God"[90] The problem is that it could be dangerous to come too close to God, "for the Lord your God is a devouring fire." The solution is that one should follow God by imitating His actions. It is explained that just as he clothes the naked, so too should we clothe the naked. Just as He visits the sick, we should do the same.[91] Equally, God comforts the mourners and buries the dead. In each instance there is a biblical example of God's action which is to be imitated. God's goodness which we should emulate includes blessing grooms, adorning the brides, visiting the sick,[92] laying *tephillin* and wearing a *tallis*.[93]

Similarly, the Torah includes commandments that we should walk in all God's ways, and that "the ways of God, [are] doing charity and justice."[94] We are instructed that we must cleave to God, we should cling to Him, and that we should serve Him. In each case we are commanded to imitate God's attributes, His character or His nature. We are to be

God-like in all our actions. Given that our task is to perfect the world, we come close to God by actively working to bring about change, in the immediate world of the community in which we live, then in the broader society and ultimately in the global community, because God saw that His creation was very very good. It is explained that the first and last letters of the Five Books of Moses spell the Hebrew word for love, and that this is a direct message that the Torah is surrounded by this primary virtue.

The Torah itself insists that the love of God cannot be separated from love of one's fellow man. We are not only made in God's image, every human life is of infinite value to God. So any act which denigrates a person is also an insult to God. The Bible states: "And now Israel, what does God require of you but to revere Him . . . and to walk in his ways."[95] From this we are told: "Just as He is gracious, so should you be gracious; just as He is merciful, you too should be merciful. Just as He is full of kindness and truth, so you too should be full of kindness and truth."[96] The importance of social or ethical action is illuminated by the response of Rabbi Hayyim of Brisk when asked the function of a rabbi. He answered unhesitatingly that the task of a rabbi is "to redress grievances of those who are abandoned and alone, to protect the dignity of the poor and to save the oppressed at the hands of the oppressor."[97]

There are two strategies which we need to take to come close to God, both of which are implicit in the statement: "But only in this should come glory: that he understands and knows Me, For I the Lord act with kindness, justice and equity in the world; For in these things I delight."[98] To understand God involves study of the Torah. To know God requires imitation of the attributes of mercy, justice, and righteousness–"He has told you, Oh man, what is good, and what the Lord requires of you: only to do justice, to love goodness, and to walk modestly with your God."[99] To fulfill this *mitzvah*, we have an obligation to engage in *gemilut hasadim*, acts of loving kindness, to reach out to our neighbors and to strangers and to work to bring about social justice.

The obligation to educate ourselves and our children is of great importance. The most basic prayer, the *Shema*, which is recited twice a day and is on the scroll cased by the *mezuzah* on the doorposts of Jewish homes, specifically reminds us that we will teach our children Torah. Learning is valued far more than material possessions or economic status. What one does to earn a living is not the key component of Jewish identity; what one knows, how one learns, and with whom one studies are far more important issues. After all, even God is said to study Torah three hours a day.[100]

When Hillel taught the Torah to the would-be convert, he did not simply state the Golden Rule. To this he added the instruction "The rest is commentary; now go and study."[101] The *Ethics of the Fathers* tells us that "The world endures because of three activities: Torah study, worship of God, and deeds of loving-kindness."[102] The Rabbis instruct us: "The following are the activities for which a person is rewarded in the World-to-Come: honoring one's father and mother, deeds of loving-kindness, and making peace between a person and his neighbor. The study of Torah, however, is as important as all of them together."[103] Study of Torah is the highest virtue because through daily Torah study we will be influenced to act consistently with the commandments therein.

JEWISH ETHICS, HUMAN RIGHTS AND DISABILITY

"If I am not for myself, who will be? And if I am only for myself, what am I?"[104]

One area of agreement between the different Jewish theologies is the centrality of ethical behavior, or the laws between man and man. *Gemilut hasadim* are positive commandments which are binding within Orthodox Judaism and for Orthodox Jews, but the intention is always that these will be universalized and that the whole world will eventually operate on principles of social justice. Given that these are laws which are essentially about the means of treating other people with dignity and respect, they are consistent with the primary ideals of human rights theory. The benefit of analyzing these commandments is that over the generations a great deal of thought has gone into the question of how to operationalise principles and how to make them realities in the day-to-day lives of us all.

It is not possible in a few short pages to survey Jewish ethics or come close to covering all the basics.[105] Instead I will attempt to capture the flavor of Jewish ethics by focusing on those principles which I think are of particular importance for people with disabilities. As such, I will explore the requirement to take action to solve social problems, the meaning of "loving one's neighbour," the concepts of justice and charity, the stumbling block principle, the rules of hospitality, the obligation to visit the sick and the requirement to watch what we say. Rabbi Katz writes that "when we observe these commandments . . . we begin to internalize the dynamics of the Torah. We become attuned to a keen sense of self, others, the universe, and, of course, God."[106]

(a) Social Responsibility

Judaism holds that each individual is responsible for both his or her own actions as well as responsible for the position which others find themselves in and the actions taken by others. We have an obligation to engage in social action and to try to better the world. In its most basic form, the principle of individual responsibility can be demonstrated by the fact that Judaism does not entertain the idea of the "innocent by-stander": "How do we know that if one sees someone drowning, mauled by beasts, or attacked by robbers, one is obligated to save him? From the verse "Do not stand by while your neighbor's blood is shed."[107] Even in circumstances where we might be nervous about acting, we have a duty to act (although not to put our own lives at risk). Clearly, then, we must be obliged to act in response to hatred or discrimination against people with disabilities which requires no bravery or drama. "Whoever can stop . . . the people of his city from sinning, but does not . . . is held responsible for the sins of the people of the city. If he can stop the whole world from sinning, and does not, he is held responsible for the sins of the whole world."[108]

The obligation is not just to intervene when we see a problem. We are required to take active measures to bring about justice. The commandment "Justice, justice you shall pursue"[109] not only refers to both just outcomes and to justice in the process of achieving the outcome. It also requires us to seek out problems and actively pursue justice. We are told that "when the community is in trouble, a person should not say 'I will go to my house and I will eat and drink and be at peace with myself.' "[110] Instead, we must respond to social needs of individuals (including people with disabilities), of segments of the community (including all Jews who are people with disabilities) as well as to the community as a whole (in the face of Anti-Semitism, for example). The mitzvah of pursuing justice should therefore protect the rights of all who are oppressed, and this clearly includes people with disabilities. Jewish theology does not permit us to sit and do nothing about injustice–we must act to remedy all abuses of human rights, including those suffered by people with disabilities.

(b) Justice not Charity

The second important ethical principle, from the perspective of the human rights of people with disabilities, is the principle of *tsedakah*–ten thought of as charity, but in fact justice. One of the biggest problems facing people with disabilities is the conceptualisation of disability being a matter of welfare, not of rights. But Jewish theology does not accept this. We are obliged to engage in acts of *tedakah* not out of the generosity of our hearts (although this is also desirable), but because justice requires that we rectify imbalances in the social and economic life of the community. Those of us who are well-positioned can not assume that we are in some way superior to those who are not. In the vernacular, we have whatever we have "by the grace of God." Therefore, we must reach out to others and bring justice into the world.

The great 12th century biblical scholar, Maimonides, taught that the highest level of *tedakah* is where we ensure the self-sufficiency and independence of the individual such that there is no longer a need for that person to have to rely on charity.[111] The examples of *tedakah* at this level are offering a person a long-term loan to establish their own business, offering a partnership in a business, or employing the person and ensuring that the salary is sufficient to keep them out of debt. Most people with disabilities are in a state of poverty because of unemployment, not because of their inability to perform the functions of the job but because they are unable to find employers who do not discriminate against them. In many cases, the person with disabilities may require some modifications to the job or to the work environment. This could be as simple as changing the width between desks to allow room for a wheelchair or the provision of readily available technology. Because it is generally believed that accommodating the needs of people with disabilities is too difficult, employers tend to avoid the problem by not offering work to people with disabilities. Jewish theology requires us to think and act differently.

The other superior levels of *tedakah* are designed to provide support to people in need in a manner which respects the dignity of the recipient. These are, in declining status, when the giver doesn't know the identity of the recipient and vice versa; when the giver knows who he gave to, but the recipient doesn't know the identity of the donor; and when the giver doesn't know the identity of the recipient, but the recipient knows the identity of the giver. In a further move to retain the dignity of a person who receives *tedakah,* that person is also obliged to give *tedakah* .[112] The amount of *tedakah* required is said to be a minimum of 10% of one's earnings (or in the case of those who avoid tax so claim to have no earnings– a sin in its own right–10% of their wealth).

The other forms of *tedakah* are giving straight to the poor, before the person even asks; giving after being asked; giving, but not enough to meet the need, or less than one is able; and giving sourly, which is still better than not giving. Although it is difficult to do, a person in need is required to ask for help. To do otherwise is to give in to one's pride. Given that the needs of people with disabilities cannot be met if others do not know what is needed, the obligation to ask for help is empowering rather than demeaning. The cost of living is much greater for people with disabilities, who may require expensive equipment or medication, than it is for others. Providing free equipment would be an ideal form of *tedakah*. Jewish communities could establish equipment pools, from which people could borrow either temporarily or permanently. This could include mobility equipment as well as computers or software, such as that which allows a blind person to use the internet. Donating equipment that is no longer needed is itself an act of *tedakah*.

The *mitzvah* of *tedakah* is considered to be one of the most important commandments, for it is through redistribution of wealth that the society becomes a more just place for all. Because in its ideal manifestation *tedakah* is about empowering people by giving them the possibility of independence and self-sufficiency, it is an essential principle for meeting the needs of all oppressed groups in society, but of overriding importance for people with disabilities for whom this is almost always an issue. Having to rely on or ask for charity is demeaning; ensuring that this is the exception, not the rule is a fundamental value of Judaism. The Talmud teaches that "*tedakah* is equal to all the other commandments combined."[113] As Telushkin comments: "this means that a just person is one who gives *tedakah*; a person who doesn't is not just mean and unjust, she is also acting illegally.[114]

(c) Loving Your Neighbor

The Golden Rule, "love your neighbor as yourself," is considered to encapsulate the essence of Judaism because it contains within its terms many of the crucial principles of Jewish theology. The biblical mandate has the additional words: "I am the Lord."[115] Rabbi Katz explains that "By loving our fellow human beings, we, as Jews, also sanctify the Will of God. That is why the Torah refers to God."[116] While it is often thought that a "neighbor" is a member of our community, or another person living in proximity to us, the Torah also tells us that God loves the stranger, and that we must treat all people with dignity and respect, neighbors and strangers alike.[117] For we were strangers in the land of Egypt. We know what it is like to be a stranger, and that we do not like to be shunned or discriminated against or hated. Hermann Cohen, a 19th century Jewish philosopher, commented: "The stranger was to be protected, although he was not a member of one's family, clan, religion, community, or people, simply because he was a human being. In the stranger, therefore, man discovered the idea of humanity."[118]

The Golden Rule is not just a feel-good *mitvah*. As always, study of the Torah provides us with the means by which this is to be carried out. First, there has been much discussion about the literal meaning of the words themselves. The Baal Shem Tov suggested a strategy regarding the words "as yourself"–"just as we love ourselves despite the faults we know we have, so should we love our neighbors despite the faults we see in them."[119] The starting point, then, is that we must love ourselves (although it may be that by extending love to others we will learn to love ourselves).

Not only must we treat all people, including people with disabilities, with great respect, but we must also not discriminate or exact revenge. We must "Let [our] fellow man's honor be as dear as [our] own."[120] Further, "we must praise others. We must care about their money just as we care about our own money and dignity. We can never derive honor from humiliating someone else."[121] People with disabilities are degraded by the use of inappropriate language–"the disabled," "cripples," "morons," "imbeciles,"–so Jews, in particular, must be sensitive to prevent such humiliation. Further, we must be aware of the way we respond to different appearances or different behaviors, with fear or repulsion, condescension or pity, and be careful to control our emotions to ensure that each person is treated with dignity.

(d) Acts of Loving Kindness

The other lessons of the Torah take the principle more broadly. The responsibility to undertake acts of loving kindness, *gemilut hasadim*, is derived from the Golden Rule: "The world stands on three things: Torah, worship of God, and doing kindness."[122] Acts of kindness include a broad range of social actions. Maimonides tells us:

> It is a positive commandment [deriving] from their words [the Talmudic Rabbis] to visit the sick, and to comfort the mourners, and to bring forth the deceased, and to lead the bride, and to escort guests, and to involve oneself with all the needs of burial, [such as]

to bear [the deceased] on one's shoulder, and to walk before him, and to eulogise, and to dig [the grave] and to bury. And similarly [one is commanded] to cause the bride and the groom to rejoice and to assist them with all their needs. And these [duties] are the Deeds of Compassion [gemilut hasadim] which are done with one's person which have no set measure. Even though all of these commandments are from their words, in fact, they are included within [the Biblical command]: "You shall love your companion as yourself"–[this means] all things which you want others to do for you, do them yourself for your brother in Torah and commandments.[123]

Of particular value to people with disabilities, who have traditionally been excluded from communities (and even from their own families), are the laws of hospitality, which signal the importance of inclusion. The Biblical account of the three angels visiting Abraham provides the content of the *mitvah*.[124] On that occasion, Abraham even puts his conversation with God on hold while he attends to the needs of the three travellers, who he does not know are on a mission from God. He greets them with humility, and immediately offers bread and water, but then provides a feast. He personally attends to their needs–setting them in the shade, washing their feet, and waiting until they have eaten before embarking on conversation. It is said that Abraham and Sarah's tent was open in four directions, so that from wherever a stranger approached they would see that they were welcome. At the time of this event, travellers depended for their survival on good will and hospitality. Today, people with disabilities do not necessarily need the food, although given the large percentage of people with disabilities living below the poverty line, this may also be the case. However, there is no doubt that many people with disabilities are isolated and alone, and the quality of life would be greatly enhanced by others reaching out and welcoming them into their homes.

The other acts of loving kindness which could have a big impact on the lives of people with disabilities relate to the law of visiting the sick. Moses prayed for the full recovery of his sister Miriam, who had a disease similar to leprosy. It is traditional, when someone is ill or undergoing surgery, to read from *Tehillim*, the Book of Psalms, which rejoices in God's goodness and virtue. Beyond praying for someone, visiting is an extremely important requirement of Jewish law. When Rabbi Akiva visited a student who was ill, he immediately set about sweeping the floor and sprinkling water. After the disciple recovered and told Rabbi

Akiva that he had revived him, Rabbi Akiva lectured "he who does not visit the sick is like a shedder of blood."[125] The sages knew that visiting is more than a social courtesy; it is therapeutic. When a person is ill they become isolated from the world, from isolation comes depression, and from depression, comes a worsening of disease. As such, what is required, as much as medicine and medical care, is human interaction. "What is needed are solace, hope, companionship, perspective, guidance, engagement, redirection, encouragement and a renewed sense of self-worth."[126]

Halacha provides guidance concerning when relatives, friends and strangers should visit the sick, and what we need to do to discharge the obligation to visit the sick. When visiting the sick we are to "pay attention to the needs of the invalid, to see what is necessary to be done for his benefit, and to give him the pleasure of one's company, also to consider his condition and to pray for mercy on his behalf."[127] Sending a card or phoning the person or the family are also valuable, but not as great as the mitzvah of visiting. While discussing death might distress an ill person, we are otherwise to ask about the condition with a view to providing whatever support we are able to. One of the worst experiences of new parents, on learning their child has an illness or disability, is the fact that they are shunned because people feel that they don't know what to say, so don't say anything. All life should be celebrated, and the need for support is even greater than usual where the problems relate to children.

(e) The Stumbling Block Principle

One final law is essential to mention. This is the law which commands: "You shall not curse the deaf and you shall not place a stumbling block before the blind. You shall fear your God"[128] and "cursed be he who misleads the blind."[129] This has been understood metaphorically–relating to giving bad advice to a person who we know will rely on that advice to their disadvantage.[130] But the literal meaning of the mitzvah is also important. In each case the victim of the action may not know the identity of the victimizer, but we are reminded that even if no man witnesses our action, God does.[131] Siegel argues that being forbidden to curse the deaf, who could not hear the curse anyway, involves a recognition that "one who suffers the impairment of a physical sense nevertheless is not unable to perceive." In other words, one should not reduce people with disabilities to their disability. It is important to acknowledge that "a physical impairment is not to be equated with a lack of intelligence or of understanding."[132]

It may also be that no one individual may be responsible for the barriers which exclude people with disabilities from society, but that we are communally responsible to remove those barriers. In the context of city development, planning which does not include such things as ramps for wheelchair users (and parents with prams), traffic lights which bleep, or Braille numbers on ATMs could literally create "stumbling blocks." All around us there are artificial barriers which interfere with the capacity of a person with disabilities to function fully in society. Combining the stumbling block principle with the obligations of social responsibility provides a strong mandate to improve the human rights of people with disabilities within Jewish theology.

CONCLUSION

Jewish theology, then, does not focus on questions of God's existence or in faith or belief in God, for these issues are considered relatively unproblematic. Instead, the focus is on the meaning of being created in God's image, and the consequences of this for our behaviour. Coming close to God is not a matter of prayer or spiritual activity, but of acting like God by being righteous, just and merciful. A crucial element of Jewish theology is the divine spark in each of us that makes us each of infinite value in our own right, and makes each of us morally equivalent to another. All life is precious, and every second of life is of indisputable worth. Every person is to be treated with dignity and respect, with the love and care we desire for ourselves. We are commanded to reach out to each other, to make each other welcome in our homes, to visit the sick, and to exercise our free will in a manner consistent with God's. We are to worship no other God–not Satan, or money, or human or supernatural heroes. We are to stand up for justice and take responsibility for the world around us. We are to share with God in the act of creation, and to perfect the world. "More than the Bible is interested in the home God made for man, it is concerned with the home man makes for God. Fundamental to it is not the natural world God created but the social world we create."[133]

Judaism has a distinct manner of understanding the world. The Jewish epistemology is that we can only know anything through the medium of Torah and that the wisdom needed to resolve current issues can be found in our sacred texts. Because the need to understand a Jewish perspective on disability is relatively new, there has been little research pulling together the relevant texts and ideas on the subject of disability. However, at the very centre of Judaism there is an approach to the world from which we can derive a Jewish perspective of disability, a perspective which is extremely supportive of the modern ideas of the human rights approach to people with disabilities.

What I have argued in this paper is that Jewish theology offers not only hope but also help to people with disabilities. We have seen that Judaism holds that we are all equal, all made in "God's image." According to Jewish theology, people with disabilities are not inherently sinful, morally degenerate or tainted in any way. People with disabilities are simply other (good or bad) people to whom bad things have happened. Further, people with disabilities should respect themselves and everybody else. They are expected, as are all Jews, to practice rituals, become righteous and give *tedakah*. "What is particularly significant is that, in any instance in the Jewish tradition, be it in the interpretation of homilies, in the description of heroes, in the legislative category, at no point is there denigration of the individual with a disability, or humor (cruel or otherwise) at the expense of this individual, or exclusion of the individual from the community as a total segregate, or a description for the handicapped individual as one who is cursed of God. . . . Disabled or not, the individual is a human being."[134]

Beyond this, I have argued that Judaism offers guidance for the way people without disabilities should treat, or behave towards, those with disabilities. First of all, people with disabilities must not be shamed or humiliated, but be treated with dignity and respect at all times. Each of us should value the lives of others, with or without disability, as we do our own. We must not make life harder for people with disabilities by "placing stumbling blocks" in their paths, and should act to remove barriers to equality of which we are aware. When people with disabilities are sick, we should visit them just as we should visit all people who are ill. We should welcome people with disabilities into our homes and show them hospitality. We should ensure that, if they are poor, people with disabilities receive the food, shelter and other support which justice demands we provide. We should ensure people with disabilities have access to education, particularly to have the opportunity to learn Torah. Overall, people with disabilities are our "neighbours" and we should treat them just as we would like to be treated.

NOTES

1. Jonathon Sacks, *Radical Then, Radical Now*, Harper Collins London (2000) at p208.

2. Jaboc Neusner, "Religion as an Account of Social Order" in *Blackwell Companion to Judaism* (2003) Blackwell, 3, at p7; Jaboc Neusner, "The Canon of Rabbinic Judaism" in *Blackwell Companion to Judaism* (2003) Blackwell, at p93-111; Neil Gillman, *Sacred Fragments* (1990) Jewish Publication Society, Philadelphia at p56, 224, David Ariel, *What Do Jews Believe* (1995) Schocken Books, NY.

3. Jonathon Sacks, *One People* (1993) Littman Library of Civilization, London. Sacks is not alone in holding this position–see for example Nathan Cardozo, (2002) *Thoughts to Ponder: Daring Observations About the Jewish Tradition* Urim Publications, New York at p153: "Beyond agreement with the foundation upon which Judaism stands Judaism is a multi-coloured tradition which encourages as many interpretations as possible." However, Reform and Conservative movements "deny certain fundamental tenets of belief that are crucial to Judaism. Once one denies them, one can no longer speak of authentic Judaism." See also Mordechai Katz, *Understanding Judaism (2000)* ArtScroll Series, Mesorah Publication, New York 2000: Different opinions about Judaism "are not really cultural diversity within Judaism, but divergence from the basic commitment of Judaism itself. . . . the key issue in divergent movements is the questioning of Torah as God's blueprint for the world," at p72-3.

4. Per Nathan Cardozo (2002) *Thoughts to Ponder: Daring Observations About the Jewish Tradition,* Urim Publications, New York at p112 See also Josephus, "Contra Ap." ii. 16 of which Kaufmann Kohler "Judaism" Jewish Encycoplaedia online <http://www.jewishencyclopedia.com/view_friendly.jsp?artid=666&letter=J> writes "Because Judaism is a system of laws and the religious doctrines only implicitly or occasionally stated, it is frequently asserted that Judaism is a theocracy, a religious legislation for the Jewish people, but not a religion."

5. *Buck v Bell* 247 US 200, 1927 at p. 207.

6. Neil Gillman, *Sacred Fragments*, Jewish Publication Society, Philadelphia, (1990) at p5.

7. *b. Shabbat 87a.*

8. References to the Talmud are most often from the Babylonian Talmud, which is generally considered to have greater application than the Jerusalem Talmud. Throughout this essay, the Babylonian Talmud is indicated with the prefix BT; the Jerusalem Talmud is indicated by the reference JT.

9. Judith Abrams, *Judaism and Disability* (1998) Gallaudet University Press, Washington DC.

10. Melinda Jones, "Judaism, Spirituality and Disability–An Australian Perspective," *Journal of Religion, Disability & Health* (2003).

11. Deuteronomy 4:2–"You shall not add to it or detract from it." Katz comments at p145 that the Torah states that anyone who wants to add or detract from the Torah is a false prophet and can be sentenced to death. Maimonides taught that belief in the unchanging nature of Torah is a basic principle of Judaism: *Thirteen Principles, Perush HaMishnayos.* Trude Weiss-Rosmarin, *Judaism and Christianity* (1997) Jonathan David, NY notes that when "[n]ew things were added to Judaism over the ages they were of one spirit, as it were, with all that preceded and succeeded them" at p19.

12. Moses Maimonides, *Mishne Torah: Hilchot Yesuda HaTorah* 2:10; *Guide to the Perplexed,* ch 58, 59 passim.

13. Kaufmann Kohler, "Judaism," Jewish Encycoplaedia online <http://www.jewishencyclopedia.com/view_friendly.jsp?artid=666&letter=J>

14. Trude Weiss-Rosmarin, *Judaism and Christianity* (1997) Jonathan David, NY at p18 attributes this interpretation to a Chassidic Rabbi.

15. Lopes Cardozo, Nathan (2000), *Judaism on Trial* ,Urim Publications, New York at p203.

16. Schopenhauer "Judaism cannot be denied the glory of being the only genuine monotheistic religion on earth; there is none beside it that possesses an objective God, the Creator of Heaven and Earth" [*Parerga and Paralipomena* 1–cited by Trude Weiss-Rosmarin, *Judaism and Christianity* (1997) Jonathan David, NY at 16].

17. Maimonides, the great medieval philosopher, states in his Code of Law that "Whosoever conceives God to be a corporeal being is a heretic and an apostate" *Mishne Torah, Hilchos Teshuvah* 3:1.

18. Adin Steinhaltz, *Simple Words* (2001) Simon & Schuster, NY at p217.

19. Lopes Cardozo, Nathan (2000), *Judaism on Trial,* Urim Publications, New York at p225. Carozo relates the comment of Rabbi Moshe Cordovero (a 16th c Kabbalist) "When your mind conceives of God, do not permit yourself to imagine that there really is a God as depicted by you, for if you do this, you will have a finite corporeal conception, God forbid. Instead your mind should dwell only on the affirmation of God's existence, and then it should *recoil*. To do more than that is to allow the imagination to reflect on God as He is Himself and such a reflection is bound to result in imaginative limitations and corporeality. Therefore put reins on your intellect and do not allow it too great a freedom, but assert God's existence and deny the possibility of comprehending Him. The mind should run to and fro–running to affirm God's existence and recoiling from any limitations, since man's imagination pursues his intellect." At 226.

20. Kaplan, Conservative, Reform, Spinoza. Rabbi Cardozo comments that "In the entire Torah there is no attempt to prove the existence of G–it is taken for granted. Nor does the Talmud. Only later thinkers under the influence of non-Jewish philosophy . . ." *Judaism on Trial* (2000) Urim Publications, New York at p224.

21. BT *Hullin* 60a.

22. Denis Prager & Joseph Telushkin (1986) *The Nine Questions People Ask About Judaism,* Touchstone Books NY at p19.

23. Genesis 17-18.

24. Numbers 11:21-23.

25. Denis Prager & Joseph Telushkin (1986) *The Nine Questions People Ask About Judaism,* Touchstone Books NY at p183.

26. See also Lopes Cardozo, Nathan (2000) *Judaism on Trial* Urim Publications New York p333.

27. Rabbi Saadia Gaon *Emunos V'Dei'os* cited by Mordechai Katz *Understanding Judaism,* ArtScroll Series, Mesorah Publication, New York (2000) at p144.

28. JT, *Haggiga* 1:7.

29. BT, *Pesahim* 50b cited by Denis Prager & Joseph Telushkin (1986) *The Nine Questions People Ask About Judaism,* Touchstone Books, NY at p19.

30. Genesis 12:1 (although Abraham had already left Ur for Canaan before the command 11:31).

31. Jonathon Sacks, *Radical Then, Radical Now* (2000) Harper Collins, London at p69.

32. Genesis 1:27.

33. Jonathon Sacks, *Radical Then, Radical Now* (2000) Harper Collins, London (2000) at p66-7.

34. Mishna, *Avot* 3:14.

35. This refers to "Who knows that your blood is redder? Perhaps his blood is redder" BT *Sanhedrin* 74a.

36. Siegel, MK, *Seminal Jewish Attitudes Toward The Handicapped* http://www. rac.org/issues/issuedr.html

37. BT *Sanhedrin 37a.*

38. Joseph Telushkin, *Jewish Literacy* (1991) William Morrow, NY at p530.

39. Alfred Kolatch, *The Second Jewish Book of Why* (1985) Jonathon David Publishers, NY, comments at 176, "Jewish tradition places the decision of who shall live and who shall die in God's hands alone. A Jew does not own her body so has no right to play with life and death."

40. Leviticus 18: 5.

41. BT, *Yoma* 85b.

42. The Life-Saving Principle (*pikuach nefesh*) is perhaps the most important of all Jewish laws, as it requires that all other Jewish laws be suspended when human life is at stake. There are 3 exceptions to this: the Commandments concerning idolatry, murder and prohibited relations.

43. Rabbi Abraham J. Heschel, cited by David Freeman & Judith Abrams, *Illness & Health in the Jewish Tradition* (1999) Jewish Publication Society, Philadelphia at p231.

44. Abraham Abraham, *The Comprehensive Guide to Medical Halachah* (1996) Feldheim Publishers, Jerusalem at p33.

45. See Fitzgerald J, "Bioethics, Disability and Death: Uncovering Cultural Bias in the Euthanasia Debate" in Jones M & Marks LAB (eds) *Disability, Divers-ability & Legal Change* (1999) Martinus Nijhoff, Dordrecht.

46. Similar issues arise in the context of prenatal testing and decisions to abort foetuses (and the Human Genome Project will provide more and more genetic markers of 'abnormality'); decisions to sterilise young women with disabilities to prevent unwanted pregnancies (rather than to prevent sexual abuse. See Jones M & Marks LAB "Valuing People through Law: Whatever Happened to Marion" in Jones M & Marks LAB (eds), *Explorations on Law & Disability in Australia,* Special Issue of Law in Context Federation Press, Sydney (2000) 147-181 and Jones M & Marks LAB, "The Dynamic Developmental Model of Emerging Rights in Children" (1994) *International Journal of Children's Rights,* Vol 2, 265-291.

47. Not only all life, but every second of every life, is invaluable: "The value of life is infinite and therefore the value of every part of it, however brief, is similarly infinite ... Once one denies the value of human life because of the nearness of death, one destroys the absolute value of all life and gives it instead a relative value only–in relation to age, health, further use to the community or any other factor one wishes to consider. The moment one is willing to shorten life by however little, the life of dying patient, on the grounds that it is of no further value, one destroys the infinite value of all human life ... Thus, even if death is near and absolutely certain, the life of a patient is still of infinite and inestimable value, and shortening it is no way different from killing an absolutely healthy individual." Per Abraham Abraham, *The Comprehensive Guide to Medical Halachah* (1996) Feldheim Publishers, Jerusalem at p193-194.

48. On this question see Rosner F., *Biomedical Ethics and Jewish Law* (2001) Ktav, New Jersey at p. 223-287; Rabbi Avi Shafran (2001) *Legalizing Assisted Suicide*

<http:// aish.com/societywork/sciencenature/Legalizing_Assisted_Suicide.asp> Bernstein S, *Doctor-Assisted Suicide* (2001) <http://aish.com/societywork/sciencenature/Doctor-Assisted_ Suicide.asp> Bernstein S, *Compassionate Murder* http://aish.com/societywork/sciencenature/Com passionate_Murder.asp Eisenberg D *End of Life Choices in Halacha* (1999) <http:// www.jlaw.com/Articles/EndofLife.html>

49. Lopes Cardozo, Nathan (2000) *Judaism on Trial,* Urim Publications, New York at p339.

50. Ecclesiastes 7:20, See also I Kings 8:46.

51. Kushner, *Living a Life that Matters* (2001) Sidgwick & Jackson, London at 52-53.

52. Lopes Cardozo, Nathan *Judaism on Trial,* (2000)Urim Publications, New York at p340.

53. Mishnah, *Avot* 2:21.

54. See Schroeder, Gerald L, *The Science of God* (1997) The Free Press, New York at p167: "Het is not something we are endowed like an unwanted inheritance or genetic defect. The norm is having goodness in the world.... Error is an aberration.... Expulsion from Eden is the 'hiding of God's face' ... With God hidden, the world assumes free reign and the potential for trouble increases."

55. Rabbi Lopes Cardozo explains that God told Noah that the cause of The Flood was robbery between men, so God was powerless to save humanity. "God informs us that He can forgive humanity when they transgress those laws which regulate the relationship between man and Himself, but He cannot forgive someone for his transgressions towards his fellow man." Lopes Cardozo, Nathan (2000) *Judaism on Trial* Urim Publications, New York at p119.

56. Proverbs 21:3.

57. Judaism does not accept the idea or "law of sin in the body." On the contrary, "God gave man sexual feelings and therefore that cannot be evil. They are neutral and depending on how man uses his sexuality, it could be positive or negative.... when husband and wife come together, the Shechina, the divine Presence, is between them!" Lopes Cardozo, Nathan (2000) *Judaism on Trial,* Urim Publications, New York at p171.

58. See Kushner HS, *Living a Life that Matters* (2001) Sidgwick & Jackson, London at p52-53.

59. Deuteronomy 30:19.

60. Schroeder, Gerald L, *The Science of God* (1997) The Free Press, New York at p174.

61. BT Berachot 5a.

62. Moses Maimonides, *Mishneh Torah*, cited by Trude Weiss-Rosmarin *Judaism and Christianity* (1997) Jonathan David, NY at p42.

63. Will Herberg, *Judaism and the Modern Man,* NY, Atheneum (1979) at p92.

64. Schroeder, Gerald L, *The Science of God* (1997) The Free Press, New York at p75-6.

65. Schroeder, Gerald L, *The Science of God* (1997) The Free Press, New York at p167.

66. Schroeder, Gerald L, *The Science of God* (1997) The Free Press, New York at p170.

67. Kolatch, Alfred J, *The Second Jewish Book of Why* (1985) Jonathon David Publishers, NY at 64; Telushkin J, *Jewish Literacy* (1991) William Morrow & Co, NY at p504.

68. Morton Siegel commented: "Further, the tradition holds that the individual with a disability represents an individuated need. This person is not a reflection of invidious progenitors. His or her disability is not the result of theodicy. It is not an affliction, nor the baneful result of transgression on the part of the parents; nor is it a matter of 'sin.' What has happened, in the technical usage of the term 'natural,' is a physiological or psychological development which is non-valuational. While the individual, accordingly, is the concern of the family, s/he is not the 'black sheep' of the family. S/he is not the albatross perched on the family tree. Today, of course, such an observation is quite gratuitous (or should be). It was much less so in ancient days." In *Seminal Jewish Attitudes Toward The Handicapped* <http://www.rac.org/issues/issuedr.html>

69. Jonathon Sacks, *Radical Then, Radical Now* (2000) Harper Collins, London at p38.

70. Schroeder, *The Science of God* (1997) The Free Press, New York at p169 (Deuteronomy 28:47; Deuteronomy 31:20; Hosea 13:6).

71. Harold S. Kushner, *When Bad Things Happen to Good People* (1981) Avon Books, NY.

72. Schroeder, Gerald L, *The Science of God* (1997) The Free Press, New York at p171.

73. Elijah, the Gaon of Vilna, *Commentary on Proverbs* 24:31, Denis Prager & Joseph Telushkin (1975) *The Nine Questions People Ask About Judaism,* Touchstone Books, NY at p65.

74. In this section I use the term Torah to refer to the entire corpus of Jewish law–both the Written Law and the Oral Law.

75. A number of the commandments cannot be complied with in the absence of the Temple.

76. This construction of Jewish law is taken from Denis Prager & Joseph Telushkin (1986) *The Nine Questions People Ask About Judaism,* Touchstone Books, NY at p48. Other scholars have divided the laws in different ways, for different purposes.

77. Denis Prager & Joseph Telushkin (1986) *The Nine Questions People Ask About Judaism,* Touchstone Books, NY at p47.

78. I consider the laws relating to visiting the sick below.

79. Isaiah, 5:16.

80. While this is true today, during the period of the 2nd Temple fine distinctions were drawn between people on the basis of disability: JT, *Haggigah* passim.

81. Telushkin J, *Jewish Literacy,* William Morrow & Co, NY (1991) at p100.

82. BT, *Yoma* 86a.

83. Nathan Lopes Cardozo (2000) *Judaism on Trial ,* Urim Publications, New York at p163. Mordechai Katz makes a similar point: "While many people have the image of a Torah-observant Jew as concerned with rituals, the observance of proper relations between human beings is equally if not more important." *Understanding Judaism,* ArtScroll Series, Mesorah Publication, New York at p154.

84. Neil Gillman (1990) *Sacred Fragments,* Jewish Publication Society, Philadelphia at p215.

85. BT, *Shabbat* 31a.

86. Leviticus 19:18.

87. Genesis 5:1.

88. JT, *Nedarim* 9:4.

89. Jonathon Sacks (2000) *Radical Then, Radical Now,* Harper Collins, London at p74.

90. Deuteronomy, 13:5.

91. BT, *Sotah* 14a.

92. Midrash, *Bereshit Rabba* 8:13.

93. *Rosh Hashana* 17b.

94. Genesis 18:19.

95. Deuteronomy 10:12.

96. BT, *Shabbat* 133b.

97. This story is recounted by Joseph B Soloveitchik, the grandson of Rabbi Hayyim of Brisk: *Halakhic Man* (1983) Jewish Publication Society of America, Philadelphia at p91.

98. Jeremiah 9:22-23.

99. Micah 6:8.

100. BT, *Avoda Zara 3b*.

101. BT, *Shabbat 31a*.

102. *Mishnah Avot 1:2*.

103. *Mishnah Peah 1:1*.

104. Hillel in *Mishnah Avot* 1:14.

105. For a more thorough grounding in this area see the writings of Rabbi Joseph Telushkin, *Jewish Wisdom,* (1994) William Morrow & Co, New York (2000) *The Book of Jewish Values* Bell Tower, New York; (2003) *The Ten Commandments of Character,* Bell Tower, New York, See also Sidney Greenberg (1996) *Words to Live By,* Jason Aronson Inc, London.

106. Mordechai Katz *Understanding Judaism,* (2000) ArtScroll Series, Mesorah Publication, New York at p157.

107. BT, *Sanhedrin 73a*.

108. BT, *Shabbat 54b*.

109. Deuteronomy 16:20.

110. BT, *Ta'anit 11a*.

111. Moses Maimonides *Mishneh Torah* "Laws Concerning Gifts to the Poor" 10:7.

112. BT, *Gitten 7b*.

113. BT, *Bava Bathra 9b*.

114. Telushkin, *Jewish Literacy* (1991) William Morrow, NY at p512.

115. Leviticus 19:18.

116. Mordechai Katz, *Understanding Judaism* (2000) ArtScroll Series, Mesorah Publication New York at p158.

117. "The stranger who resides with you . . . you shall love him as yourself, for you were strangers in the land of Egypt: I am the Lord your God" Leviticus 19:34.

118. Cited by Telushkin, J *The Book of Jewish Values* (2000) Bell Tower, New York.

119. Recounted by Mordechai Katz, *Understanding Judaism* (2000) ArtScroll Series, Mesorah Publication, New York at p158.

120. *Mishnah Avot 2:15*.

121. Moses Maimonides, *Mishneh Torah*, Hilchos Dei'os 6:3.

122. *Mishnah Avot 1:2*.

123. BT, *Sota 14a*, Moses Maimonides *Laws of Human Character*.

124. Genesis 18 v2-8.

125. BT, *Nedarim 40a*.

126. David Freeman & Judith Abrams *Illness & Health in the Jewish Tradition* (1999) Jewish Publication Society, Philadelphia at pxxi.

127. Code of Jewish Law, CXCIII:87, "Laws Concerning Visiting the Sick."

128. Leviticus 19:14.

129. Deuteronomy 27:18.

130. BT, *Sifra* discussed by Telushkin, *Book of Jewish Values* at p158.

131. Telushkin *Book of Jewish Values* (2000) Bell Tower NY at p86.

132. Morton K. Siegel, *Seminal Jewish Attitudes Toward the Handicapped* <http://www.rac.org/issues/issuedr.html>

133. Jonathon Sacks, *Radical Then, Radical Now* (2000) Harper Collins, London (2000) at p71.

134. Morton K. Siegel, *Seminal Jewish Attitudes Toward the Handicapped* <http://www.rac.org/issues/issuedr.html>

doi: 10.1300/J095v10n03_08

"L'Dor v'Dor,"
From Generation to Generation: One Community's Response to Jewish Genetic Diseases

Becca Hornstein, BS

SUMMARY. Most American Jews are of Ashkenazic (Eastern European) descent and, as such, are at risk of being carriers of one or more Jewish genetic diseases. There is a compelling need to educate teens and young adults about these diseases, inheritance patterns, genetic counseling and screening before they have children. To overcome the barriers of the high costs of testing and concerns about the loss of confidentiality, the Jewish community in Phoenix, Arizona has created an affordable screening and genetics education program to reach out to rabbis, physicians, and Jewish individuals. doi:10.1300/J095v10n03_09 *[Article copies available for a fee from The Haworth Document Delivery Service: 1-800-HAWORTH. E-mail address: <docdelivery@haworthpress.com> Website: <http://www.HaworthPress.com> © 2006 by The Haworth Press, Inc. All rights reserved.]*

Becca Hornstein is Executive Director, Council For Jews With Special Needs, Inc., 12701 North Scottsdale Road, Suite 205, Scottsdale, AZ 85254-5453 (E-mail: becca@cjsn.org).

[Haworth co-indexing entry note]: " 'L'Dor v'Dor,' From Generation to Generation: One Community's Response to Jewish Genetic Diseases." Hornstein, Becca. Co-published simultaneously in *Journal of Religion, Disability & Health* (The Haworth Pastoral Press, an imprint of The Haworth Press, Inc.) Vol. 10, No. 3/4, 2006, pp. 147-153; and: *Jewish Perspectives on Theology and the Human Experience of Disability* (ed: Rabbi Judith Z. Abrams, and William C. Gaventa) The Haworth Pastoral Press, an imprint of The Haworth Press, Inc., 2006, pp. 147-153. Single or multiple copies of this article are available for a fee from The Haworth Document Delivery Service [1-800-HAWORTH, 9:00 a.m. - 5:00 p.m. (EST). E-mail address: docdelivery@haworthpress.com].

Available online at http://jrdh.haworthpress.com
doi:10.1300/J095v10n03_09

KEYWORDS. Jewish, genetic diseases, genetic screening, community education, inherited disabilities

In the finest tradition of Jewish mothers everywhere, I take great pleasure in passing down the religious traditions, cherished books, Yiddish phrases and my grandmother's recipes for matzah balls and chopped liver to my children. As an Ashkenazi Jew (of Eastern European descent), I'm afraid there are other things that may be inherited, and those are Jewish genetic diseases.

The vast majority of American Jewish families are of Eastern European (Ashkenazi) descent and, therefore, are at increased risk of inheriting dozens of genetic diseases which are more prevalent among Ashkenazi Jews. Most Jewish adults do not know that one in 25 Ashkenazi Jews is a carrier of the Tay-Sachs gene and that, if both parents of a newborn are carriers of the defective gene, there is a 25% chance that the baby will be afflicted with this fatal disease. Likewise, one in 25 Ashkenazi Jews is a carrier of the Cystic Fibrosis gene; one in 9 is a carrier of the gene for Gaucher Disease. It is time to increase awareness of these diseases in our Jewish communities and to encourage screening of Jewish young adults who may be unaware of these diseases, their genetic character and the availability of screening tests to determine carrier status.

In the past, rabbis typically included a few words about testing for Tay-Sachs disease when they met with a couple in preparation for their wedding and marriage, and many Jewish communities held annual screening events for Tay-Sachs disease at which the test was available for around $25. Today, outside of the Orthodox communities, most Jewish young adults are unaware of this risk and paying for genetic screening has become too expensive for the average young adult.

While the current high rate of intermarriage between Jews and non-Jews dilutes the gene pool and lowers the risk of having a child with one of the Jewish genetic diseases, it does not eradicate the problem. Those diseases that are considered "Jewish genetic diseases" exist in non-Jews as well although at a different frequency rate. Cystic Fibrosis occurs at the same frequency rate among Caucasians in the U.S. Thus, a Jewish woman and her non-Jewish husband may still both be carriers of the defective gene that causes Cystic Fibrosis.

A demographic study commissioned by the Jewish Federation of Greater Phoenix in 2000 said that there are approximately 83,000 Jews in my community. In a large Ashkenazi Jewish population screened for carrier status for the nine most prevalent Jewish genetic diseases, 15% (1:7) will be positive for one or more of these diseases. In 2002, my agency collaborated with several other Jewish organizations to educate and screen young Jewish adults.

PHASE I–
DISTRIBUTION OF EDUCATIONAL MATERIALS TO RABBIS AND PHYSICIANS

In September of 2002, the Council For Jews With Special Needs distributed to community rabbis and physicians a pamphlet entitled "What You Should Know About . . . Jewish Genetic Diseases" that was prepared by the National Foundation for Jewish Genetic Diseases in New York City. In addition, they received "A Brief Guide to Jewish Genetic Diseases" and a list of local genetic counseling facilities and laboratory information for Ashkenazi Jewish carrier testing that could be copied and given to the young adults who visit rabbis and physicians.

A follow-up survey to those who received this material indicated that more needed to be done to educate the Jewish community about this serious concern. Jewish Family & Children's Services, Jewish Federation's Young Leadership Division and the Shalom Healing Center of Temple Chai joined the Council For Jews With Special Needs to form the "Greater Phoenix Jewish Genetic Diseases Project Committee."

PHASE II–
COMMUNITY PRESENTATIONS ON JEWISH GENETIC DISEASES

The committee spent a year researching how other Jewish communities are addressing the need for genetic disease awareness and carrier screening. We were surprised to learn that very few Jewish communities offer screening, and so we had to create our own model. (In the very observant Orthodox communities, teens are tested in their private schools. The community retains the screening results to be referenced only when young people are introduced in anticipation of possible marriage-matches. This has proven highly effective at lowering the births of children with Jewish genetic diseases.)

Before the screening could take place, committee members developed a power point presentation on Jewish genetic diseases and carrier testing. That presentation was then marketed to all of the synagogues, religious schools, youth groups, young adult groups, university student organizations and community service groups.

The power point presentation also focused on educating the public about genetic diseases and carrier rates for autosomal recessive inheritance. Each of the nine most prevalent diseases was described, along with information about genetic screening and counseling. On average, the power point presentation along with questions and answers took 45 minutes.

PHASE III–
EDUCATIONAL AND SCREENING EVENT

At the same time that work was being done to produce and deliver the power point presentations, committee members were seeking competitive bids from various labs to get reduced rates for carrier testing. The goal was to offer testing for the four most prevalent genetic diseases (Tay-Sachs, Canavan, Cystic Fibrosis and Familial Dysautonomia) at a rate much lower than the usual cost of $1,000–$1,400 if privately paid. If the cost could be significantly lowered, the committee hoped that by raising funds locally, we could subsidize the difference and offer the test panel for four diseases at a cost of $36 per person.

After exhaustive research, we were able to develop a relationship with a lab that agreed on a discounted rate for the testing. Through the generosity of many community donors and foundations, the committee raised $66,000 to pay for the expenses incurred by this project and for subsidizing the individual carrier tests.

Marketing for the Screening Event was targeted only within the Jewish community. Since this was the first time in over 25 years that testing for Jewish genetic diseases was being offered, there was concern that the response might exceed the committee's ability to subsidize testing for young adults.

The committee was very careful about having the "informed consent" document reviewed by an attorney. The geneticist and genetics counselors on the committee reviewed all questionnaires related to medical and family history. The lab providing the testing worked closely with the committee to assure that all necessary background information would be gathered and accompany the blood samples to the lab. This project required a precise and secured "paper trail."

To insure that everyone who was tested was truly giving "informed consent," all participants were required to attend either one of the community (power point) presentations, the panel discussion at the screening event or a power point presentation on the day of the screening. Participants could not meet with a genetics counselor and then have blood drawn until they had listened to a presentation.

The education and screening event began with a 90-minute panel presentation. Dr. Kirk Aleck, a geneticist with St. Joseph's Hospital and Medical Center, explained autosomal recessive inheritance and gave information about specific Jewish genetic diseases. Dr. Ann Bogle, a genetic counselor, explained about the role of a genetic counselor. Dr. Joel Gereboff, chairman of the Jewish Studies Department of Arizona State University, talked about traditional and contemporary Jewish views on genetic testing. The presentations were followed by a question and answer period. Upon the completion of the panel presentation, participants were directed to meet briefly with a genetic counselor before signing all consent forms and proceeding to be tested.

More than 200 adults from the Phoenix area as well as from other cities and states attended the event; 134 individuals were tested. The cost for testing was $36 for the basic panel of tests for carrier screening for Tay-Sachs, Canavan, Cystic Fibrosis, and Familial Dysautonomia. Individual tests to screen for other Ashkenazic genetic diseases such as Bloom Syndrome, Gaucher Disease, Fanconi Anemia, Niemann-Pick Disease, and Mucolipidosis IV were offered at a discounted rate as well.

Since the target audience was Jewish adults of childbearing age, the basic panel of tests was offered at $36 for adults ages 18-45. Anyone over the age of 45 years old was asked to pay $250 for that panel of tests to insure that we did not deplete our funds intended for subsidized testing.

One of the significant selling points of this event was that the test results would be completely confidential. Each participant would be advised of the results; it would not be processed through their insurance company. They could decide whether or not to share the information with their primary physician or family members.

Dr. Kirk Aleck, a geneticist, provided guidance on all medical issues. Within a few weeks, Dr. Aleck or one of several genetic counselors made personal phone calls to all of those participants who tested positive for being a carrier for one of the diseases. Participants who tested positive for being a carrier of one of the genes for a Jewish genetic disease were then offered information about genetic counseling. Those whose tests were negative received a letter from Dr. Aleck with the results. A follow-up survey was included in all of the mailings to help the committee evaluate the project.

Test results	# of Positive Carriers
Canavan Disease	6/134
Cystic Fibrosis	7/134
Familial Dysautonomia	4/134
Tay-Sachs Disease	4/134
Gaucher Disease	1/42
Bloom Syndrome	0/18
Fanconi Anemia	0/18
Niemann-Pick Disease	0/18
Mucolipidosis IV	0/18

In summary, 21 of 134 participants (16%) were found to be carriers. One individual was a carrier for two diseases.

The following year, the committee held its second annual event. In April of 2006, the education and screening event was held at a Jewish Community Center in Chandler, Arizona, which is in closer proximity to the students who attend Arizona State University and the growing community of young Jewish adults in Phoenix's "East Valley." The format of the day was changed only slightly to accomodate a more streamlined delivery of the educational presentation, meeting with genetic counselors and blood draws.

Seventy-four young adults were screened for the basic panel of four diseases. Fourteen individuals tested positive as carriers of the genetic mutation for Tay-Sachs, Canavan, Cystic Fibrosis or Familial Dysautonomia. On this occassion, one couple both received positive results on the Tay-Sachs screening, and they were immediately referred for genetic counseling.

FUTURE PLANS FOR THIS PROJECT

Based on the success of the 2005 and 2006 education and screening events, the committee applied for a grant from the Greater Phoenix Jewish Community Foundation to partially fund screening events for the next three years. Committee members continue to seek private donations and hope to establish an endowment fund that will provide the necessary financial resources for future screening events. The committee has also applied to become an independent non-profit agency with 501 (c) 3 status.

In an effort to distribute educational material in the most efficient and up-to-date manner, the project committee plans to produce both a booklet and a DVD with all of the educational and religious information on it. The committee chairpersons are also engaged in a dialogue with other cities that have held Jewish genetic diseases screenings. They hope to establish a national consortium to create replicable programs for communities of all sizes.

In recognition of the impact of this project on the Phoenix-area Jewish community, the Jewish Federation of Greater Phoenix awarded the project its *Belle Latchman Community Service Award* in December of 2006. The committee has re-named the education and screening project "*L'Dor v'Dor*: From Generation to Generation." There is much of value to be handed down from grandparents to parents to their children, but what better gift from one generation to another than the gift of knowledge.

doi: 10.1300/J095v10n03_09

Executive Summary:
Minneapolis Jewish Community
Inclusion Program for People with Disabilities
Research Report

Claire Buchwald, PhD

SUMMARY. The Chasidic master Yehudi HaKadosh said, "Good intentions alone not accompanied by action are without value. The main thing is the action, as this is what makes the intention so profound." The Minneapolis Jewish community, committed to respond to the needs of Jews with disabilities and their families, conducted a research study to

---

This was a report prepared for the Minneapolis Jewish Federation, the Minneapolis Jewish Community Center, the Jewish Family and Children's Service and members of the community. For more information on the Minneapolis Jewish Community Inclusion Program for People with Disabilities, contact the Community Inclusion Office at 952-542-4838. This program is supported by a generous grant from both the Jay and Rose Phillips Family Foundation and the Jewish Community Foundation of the Minneapolis Jewish Federation.

Claire Buchwald, PhD, is Researcher and Report Author. She is Director of the Focus Interaction Research.

This Research Report was commissioned by The Minneapolis Jewish Federation, Jewish Family and Children's Service of Minneapolis, Sabes Jewish Community Center.

Permission is granted from Shelly Christensen, MA, Program Manager, Jewish Community Inclusion Program for People with Disabilities, 13100 Wayzata Boulevard, Suite 400, Minnetonka, MN 55305 (E-mail: Schristensen@jfcsmpls.org).

[Haworth co-indexing entry note]: "Executive Summary: Minneapolis Jewish Community Inclusion Program for People with Disabilities Research Report." Buchwald, Claire. Co-published simultaneously in *Journal of Religion, Disability & Health* (The Haworth Pastoral Press, an imprint of The Haworth Press, Inc.) Vol. 10, No. 3/4, 2006, pp. 153-181; and: *Jewish Perspectives on Theology and the Human Experience of Disability* (ed: Judith Z. Abrams and William C. Gaventa) The Haworth Pastoral Press, an imprint of The Haworth Press, Inc., 2006, pp. 153-181. Single or multiple copies of this article are available for a fee from The Haworth Document Delivery Service [1-800-HAWORTH, 9:00 a.m. - 5:00 p.m. (EST). E-mail address: docdelivery@haworthpress.com].

Available online at http://jrdh.haworthpress.com

identify specific needs so that the response would be effective. Participants in the research included Jews with disabilities, family members, rabbis and other community professionals. It became clear that the good intentions of the institutions were not enough to help Jews with disabilities move from invisibility to visibly. The research moved the community to action and became the foundation for our innovative and successful Jewish Community Inclusion Program for People with Disabilities. doi:10.1300/J095v10n03_11 *[Article copies available for a fee from The Haworth Document Delivery Service: 1-800-HAWORTH. E-mail address: <docdelivery@haworthpress.com> Website: <http://www.HaworthPress.com>*

KEYWORDS. Inclusion, community action, disability, Judaism, research

INTRODUCTION

The people who shared their time and experiences in this research say poignant things:

If a parent doesn't stay on top of everything twenty-*five* hours a day, it can be a disaster. A parent has to dot every "i" and cross every "t" or she is lost. I cannot depend on anybody in this community to work with me for my daughter unless I'm in charge of every detail from beginning to end.

After my daughter was born, I had no positive experiences in the Jewish community. I felt very alienated. People didn't know how to respond to me.

I lost my business and almost lost my house when my son was diagnosed. [Religious school] had nothing for people with special needs in those days. The kids who knew my son from school teased him and he'd react. Yet he wanted to go there. How many kids that age are so eager to go to Hebrew school? We got one of those "In all my years, your kid is the worst" speeches from the director at the time. A teacher said she was scared of my son. And he just wanted to go to religious school.

Lack of physical access to buildings has been a problem for me. It's hard to be involved if you can't even get in the door!

Some people . . . were not nice to me because they didn't know what my disability was. As I got older, people became more and more nasty. I didn't feel like I belonged there.

I hated camp! They pulled my mom aside to talk about a very embarrassing problem. It was right in front of me and my best friend. I was crying and upset and they just kept talking about this problem I was really trying hard to get over. They told my best friend to shut up. I was still crying.

I told my Mom, "I have two disabilities: one physical and one being Jewish." . . . Why is the Jewish community not as welcoming [of people with disabilities] as the Christian community? For years, I have been living in a Christian world. I go to Christian activities, Easter parties. My Christian friends have groups with pastors and priests, but there are no Jewish groups for me.

Jewish people are supposed to be compassionate and understanding, yet I always felt that people meeting my child in the community were more times than not uncomfortable with who she was. They stayed at a distance, were very peripheral. She was never really accepted; she was always kept on the fringe of things.

When a parent has a "typical" child, ultimately, in the backs of our minds, we say to ourselves "This too shall pass" and "If I keep sending the right messages to my children, it's going to be okay." When you are a parent of a child with a special need or developmental disability, you never ever have one moment in raising that child where you can step back and say, "Ultimately, it will be okay"; or "This too shall pass." You never have that peace of mind . . . You always feel you have to be on-guard or on alert 24 hours a day . . . It sits in your mind and on your heart forever. It's frightening if you don't have people in your community working with you and recognizing that this is your gift from God forever, reassuring you that your child will be in this community for her/his whole life and that the community will be a partner in taking care of that person. We wonder what will happen when we're older and don't have the energy, or when we need assistance ourselves, or when we die. A parent is thinking about these issues every day from the time their child is a baby. They can never just know that this too will be okay.

These are the truths of the life experiences of people with disabilities and their families and, even so, they are only splinters of their experiences in all their complexity.

Program directors and other professionals have their truths, too, truths that may not be as moving but are just as real to them in their earnest desire to serve the community.

> We have signs about hearing aids and signers (though we have had almost no request for that). We hand out materials on Saturday mornings giving information about how we can help; we can even meet people at the door, but not everyone wants to work with us on these areas.

> We want to include people with disabilities, but we want to do so appropriately. It would be a shame to say "Come in, come in!" and then not be able to meet people's needs . . . We need to gear up in some areas before we can welcome people with disabilities and know we will have the right resources for them.

> Our strength and our greatest need is how to build a partnership with families . . . There are often mixed messages from parents. On the one hand, they want special handling–special attention and adaptations for their kids. On the other hand, they want their kid to be like every other kid.

> People don't realize how much money inclusion work costs. They think that the Federation has limitless money, that it should not only meet all the many inclusion needs within the community while continuing to meet everyone else's needs, but also reach out to people with disabilities beyond the Jewish community. The Federation cannot do everything everyone thinks it can.

> We have an autistic kid in one of our classrooms. This child came to us with such little developmental background. He didn't know basic concepts, like shapes or what day of the week it was when his peers were already reading and doing arithmetic. It was very hard for the teachers. How can she include him? He is at a totally

different level in everything. He moves around during class; he can't focus–and he is not the only child with a special need in the classroom.

When I look at serving 150 kids and I have to spend an extra $125 for a bus, just for one trip, just for one student or use it to transport 50 kids, how can I decide? We want to be inclusive, but we also have very limited funds. It is difficult as a nonprofit, especially one that is not subsidized by the government, to serve all students well.

We have a problem with knowing when and where to draw lines–what we think is best for the child and what parents say they want are not always the same thing. Sometimes, we think parents sell their kids short or expect too much for them or want things for them that we cannot provide. We need a third party or an assessment, but parents aren't always willing to get one. Do we just do what they want? Do we just do what we think is best? Is there a point at which we tell them that their kid cannot attend until he or she has been assessed? There are a host of legal and ethical issues here.

Overnight camps have a problem in that parents of kids with special needs want to send their kids with advocates or appropriate staff assigned to them. At the same time, those without special needs are ready for a freer, more grown-up camping experience, which they can't have when there ends up being seven adults to 10 kids. As a result of the imbalance of staff to students, some students [especially those without disabilities] don't want to take part any more.

There have been times in our nursery school program when we just didn't have the right environment for a student with special needs– St. David's is better equipped to handle children with disabilities–especially in terms of trained staff.

There are so many needs and expectations in educational settings as it is. For example, at the Jewish Day schools, they are already stretched, and dealing with special needs is often especially hard.

As we read the two sets of truths above–the lived experience of exclusion or lack of support and the lived experience of trying to stretch limited resources to balance and serve the needs of large, diverse populations–we become aware of the difficulties that face any community as it approaches complex, multi-faceted issues like inclusion. We realize, too, that a faith community takes on higher expectations and standards than some other communities. How we run our organizations, who we include, how people are treated, which values we exemplify, all become major questions that reflect on ourselves as individuals, groups, and a people. It is easy, especially at this time in history, to agree that all members and potential members of our community are important, that everyone should be respected, served, valued, and fully included. No one would disagree with this interviewee's statement: "We need to think differently, to realize that Jewish people [with disabilities] are people first. They are not disabled people, but *people* with disabilities." Still, we must recognize that, as impatient–and rightfully so–as many people are for change, it will take time. It will take fundraising and reallocation of money. It will take continued persistence and vision. It will take action not from a few but from many.

Three major themes emerge from this research:

1. *The Jewish community needs inclusion.* We need it to uphold several Jewish values emphasized by respondents: *Ahavat Israel* (love of fellow humans/Jews), *Rachmanut* (compassion) and *Chesed* (loving kindness/loyalty–how one treats others). We need it so that we do not lose members of our community. We need it because it can help us develop as individuals and as a community, to move past our own prejudices, fears, and limitations. We need it the way we need all the different personalities and abilities among us. People with disabilities can be some of our strongest leaders, our kindest souls, our most gifted artists, our bravest examples, our most lovely neighbors, our favorite friends, our most exhilarating students, our most loyal congregants, our most responsible associates, our most resourceful teachers, our most loving family members, our most dependable employees, our most tireless volunteers, our most inspiring peers, our very best.

Here are just a handful of examples of extraordinary people who took part in the research, people the Jewish community will retain through inclusion or lose through lack of inclusion. One mother who was interviewed found a way for her child to be brought into social interaction by teaching him, with photographs she attached to sticks, to match the names and faces of his classmates. Another founded support groups for people with children with disabilities. Another wrote an article that, overnight, made hundreds of people within the Jewish community aware of the need to serve and include people with developmental disabilities. Still another has become a professional in the field, first working as a teacher at her daughter's school and then developing a major effort to make it possible for all Jewish children to receive a Jewish education. These parents are inspiring in their dedication, initiative, persistence, creativity, and drive. An adolescent with cerebral palsy, who despite the teasing he continues to face, earnestly intends to "make the world a better place" provides an example for us of goodness and positive energy. A former engineer with a traumatic brain injury demonstrates courage and an admirable skill for putting people at ease when she uses gentle humor to describe how she became injured. As one meets people in the community with disabilities and their families, it becomes clear not only what the Jewish community could do for them but even more so what a startling array of gifts, values, and strengths the community will lose without them.

2. *We need to move from "them versus us" thinking to attain a richer "us."* It is undeniably true that full inclusion is expensive in terms of time and money. Still, the same could be true about inclusion of anyone. Should Jews be given all the same rights and benefits in the U.S. or Minnesota, even though most original settlers were Christian? Of course we believe that Jews should be full members of the larger society, just as we theoretically believe that the Minneapolis Jewish community should serve all its members, not just those without disabilities. We need to remember that belief when it comes to allocating money. Every person counts. As one participant pointed out, instead of dividing things up by saying that it would cost x amount to serve people without disabilities and x + y if we want to include those with disabilities, we should look at total program cost (just the way we do when we draw up budgets for programs that offer scholarships) to serve *all* potential participants. As we do so, we will gain a less divisive approach that can benefit our community in more than one way. Since each of us is potentially a person with a disability (or some other difference that could be pointed to–a person who is more or less artistic, more or less verbal, male or female, taller or shorter, Ashkenazic or Sephardic, darker or paler, interfaith or single-faith, well or sick, more or less observant), the changes we make to move from divisiveness to inclusion will potentially benefit each of us directly and our community as a whole.

3. *Finally, recognize that each person and each organization has a role to play.* Inclusion will not happen just from wishing and waiting for others–the leaders, Federation, big synagogues, the government,

wealthy families–to take action. It is incumbent on every one of us to promote inclusion, and it is possible for each one of us to make a difference. It is for this reason that we have divided and arranged the recommendations into lists of actions and specific agents in the section following the executive summary. There is a list of recommendations of what each individual, organization or synagogue, and rabbi can do, as well as what the Federation and the Inclusion Program can do, to promote inclusion. Some of these recommendations cost little or nothing to implement; some can be done right away. The process of inclusion needs to be wide-scale and ongoing, but each individual can make a significant contribution.

BACKGROUND

Members of the Jewish community of Minneapolis wish to ensure that our community welcomes all potential participants in Jewish life and includes every person fully. To this end, several people have worked hard over the last several years to initiate a community-wide inclusion[1] process to include people with disabilities[2] in our community. In 2000, the Minneapolis Jewish community received a generous three-year grant from the Jay and Rose Phillips Family Foundation to bring existing efforts together, form a central coordinating office for a community-wide inclusion program, determine what the community needs to do in order to become inclusive, and set out to work towards those goals. The grant work is a joint effort of the Minneapolis Jewish Federation (Federation), Jewish Family and Children's Services (JFCS), and the Minneapolis Jewish Community Center (JCC).

RESEARCH DESIGN AND GOALS

This report provides the results of the research that was conducted in the spring and early summer of 2001. The research was intended as a needs assessment to guide the early stages of the inclusion program. The study was performed by an independent consultant, FOCUS Interactive Research, who worked with the Community Inclusion Coordinator and was guided by the Inclusion Program Research Advisory Committee. The research consisted of three components: a mailed survey; a building accessibility assessment carried out by individual organizations; and a process of in-depth interviews and focus groups.

SUMMARY OF RECOMMENDATIONS FROM THE STUDY

- Make sure that people with disabilities and their families are represented in all areas of the inclusion program and on all other committees.
- Build a long-term process with momentum, substantive changes, positive feeling, and real action without delay.
- Recognize that money is essential in order to make important aspects of inclusion possible. Make finding, raising, and allocating that money a priority.
- Organize, staff, and support a central Inclusion Office. Staff in that office can: compile and share information, keep the community focused on inclusion, assist with communication, link and support organizations and individuals, arrange events and activities, advise committees, advocate on behalf of people with disabilities, help raise money, and be a first-call-for-help and referrals related to disability.
- Create a centralized resource (within the Inclusion Office) that contains information about individuals with disabilities who choose to participate so that they or their parents do not have to repeat everything about themselves and their disability each time they want to take part in a class, program, or activity or each time there is staff turnover.
- Publicize resources effectively.
- Educate people at all levels and all ages about disabilities, about Jewish values that support inclusion.
- Train staff members in every position at every Jewish organization about disability.
- Make all buildings in the Jewish community fully accessible.
- Be inclusive at every age in educational, social, and recreational programs.
- Look beyond immediate concerns of one synagogue, school, or denomination to serve everyone in an inclusive way.
- Education directors, rabbis and other leaders need to provide moral leadership for inclusion.
- Leaders throughout the Jewish community–in synagogues, on boards, in lay leadership positions, in the clergy, and on staff–need to demonstrate commitment to inclusion through positive attitude and example.
- Attitude change is essential. Promote positive attitudes: foster values that support empathy, inclusiveness, supportiveness, respect,

recognition of individuality, and emphasis on ability rather than disability.

- Support parents of children with disabilities.
- Create opportunities for people with disabilities to teach, lead, serve, work in, and be part of the community.
- Perform networking and outreach to serve the greatest number of people with disabilities as completely and effectively as possible.
- Major community institutions, particularly Federation, need to commit money (both start-up and ongoing), organize efforts, and develop leadership, in order for inclusion efforts to succeed.
- Provide better and more frequent transportation to events, services, activities, and religious schools. Transportation is a major issue for many people with disabilities.
- Promote community involvement, volunteerism, and direct action by individuals focused on inclusion.
- Serve children by expanding educational services in our schools and synagogues.
- Serve teens and young adults by providing more social opportunities, more educational opportunities, inclusion in camps and trips, and better transportation.
- Serve adults with disabilities by offering companionship, dating services, social activities, and transportation. Be aware that some adults with disabilities desire the opportunity to be with others who have similar disabilities.
- Meet a key need of adults and their families by creating Jewish housing options for adults with disabilities.
- Other programs, services, and changes that community members are requesting include: Jewish support groups (at secular institutions, like Courage Center and within the community); volunteers to accompany Jewish people with disabilities to community activities; assistance with swimming and using the gym; ASL interpreters, audio devices, and real-time captioning; options for non-mainstream programs; greater sensitivity; and emphasis on educational issues.

SUMMARY OF RESEARCH RESULTS

Mail Survey

The survey was designed by the Research Advisory Committee with assistance from Jeff Priest, a Research Associate at the Institute on Community Integration at the University of Minnesota. It was mailed to all households on the Federation mailing list. The survey responses show us that all areas of inclusion are important to respondents, as are services specifically designed for people with disabilities. The most frequent wishes expressed are for: attitude change; more education and awareness-raising; greater physical accessibility to buildings; more ASL interpreting and other services for the deaf or hearing-impaired; and services for the elderly. Respondents who took part in the mail survey, the one-on-one interviews, and the focus groups all made similar and overlapping suggestions. These suggestions have been organized by category and then summarized into recommendations to be found in this Executive Summary and the Actions and Agents sections of the report.

Building Accessibility Training

In June of 2001, the Research Advisory Committee organized a training workshop on how to perform a building accessibility survey. The workshop was taught by Margot Imdieke Cross from the Minnesota State Council on Disability. The workshop was open to all organizations and programs within the Minneapolis Jewish community. Each was encouraged to send at least one designated representative, such as a building supervisor, who would be in charge of the physical accessibility survey at the institution's building or the building that housed the program. Representatives from 18 community institutions attended the training.

The training met the goal of providing information and tools to Jewish community organizations so that they could evaluate their building's physical accessibility. It also began the long-term work involved in meeting our other two goals: gauging the physical accessibility of the Minneapolis Jewish community overall and looking to the future in terms of what individual organizations and the community as a whole need to do in order to achieve full inclusion.

Because the community is involved in a capital campaign which will result in significant upgrading of accessibility in many of our institutions, the accessibility study will be updated at the conclusion of the new construction.

Focus Groups and Interviews

Positive Experiences

For many, that the most positive thing they can say about their experiences in the Minneapolis Jewish community is that they believe the recent developments, including the initiation of this project, are good. Education, Inclusion, and B'nai Mitzvah programs have also been praised. So has the JCC's inclusive summer camp and Inclusion Coordinator. Some people note positive change and hope concerning Talmud Torah's programs with its new director and collaboration with the Sha'arim[3] program. Everyone who has been involved with Sha'arim speaks of it in glowing terms. Those who have been involved in advocacy or support groups, such as inclusion groups or Lech Lecha,[4] say that their involvement and discussions with others have been positive experiences for them.

Positive Attitudes and Values

Participants say that there is support for inclusion in Jewish theology, though it is often not practiced as a value. Respondents report that people in several programs and organizations in the Jewish community have been caring, though they often have not had the knowledge, money, or other resources to be successful in their efforts at education or inclusion of people with disabilities.

Negative Experiences

Physical barriers. Not being able to get into a synagogue or sanctuary or up to a bimah; not being able to attend classes or youth groups or take part in field trips; not being able to get transportation to evening events or Torah study.

Difficulties in educational, camp, and youth group settings. Teachers and counselors who do not know how to work with or include children with disabilities; daily calls to parents about their children; being asked to leave a religious school program because of their children's special needs; mean words or actions of children; disrespectful, fearful comments by staff; invitations to participate without any real efforts at integrating special needs students into a class or group; lack of opportunity to attend overnight camps or take part in youth group activities.

Dearth of companionship. Not being able to find members of the Jewish community (with or without special needs) to accompany people to activities; not being able to connect with Jewish peers (children and adults) who have similar disabilities; need for a dating service for Jews with disabilities; lack of big brothers/sisters for kids with special needs.

Lack of inclusion in religious services or activities. Reactions of fear or disgust; being ignored rather than welcomed; being asked to leave because people made noises caused by their disability; not being allowed to have a Bar/Bat Mitzvah, because "it wouldn't be fair to the other kids"; not being supported or encouraged or tutored enough to take an active part in services.

Absence of good programs or services. Jewish education (all ages); Bar/Bat Mitzvah preparation; teen social experiences; adult social opportunities; family activities that are inclusive of people with disabilities; Jewish group homes or assisted living options; high-quality vocational education; transportation for people who use wheelchairs.

Perception of lack of support by leaders and funders. Experiences with rabbis and agency staff who were uninformed or unsupportive; perception that Federation makes practically everyone a priority but people with disabilities.

Negative Attitudes and Values

Participants mention that, while some members of congregations and schools are openly hostile, more often they are simply indifferent or unwelcoming. The high value placed on school achievement, financial success, marriage and child-bearing in the Jewish community, some or all of which may not apply to people with disabilities, tend to marginalize people. One participant summarizes, "There is so much denial, shame, and wanting to look good here. There's the attitude that all Jewish kids are gifted and talented; we don't have disability—or any problem—in our community." Similarly, some people feel that the emphasis put on education in Jewish culture creates an environment in which children with cognitive disabilities in particular are seen as non-entities. Parents of people with disabilities say that their children have been treated with disrespect by peers and sometimes educators, or, even when they have been treated decently, they have not been embraced as friends or full participants

Models and Resources Include:

The St. Paul JCC; some churches, including St. Stephen's Catholic Church and Plymouth Congregational Church; the Community Integration department at the University of Minnesota; PACER; ARC; St. David's School; Jewish communities and organizations elsewhere (including in Rockville, Maryland; Phoenix, Arizona; the Chicago area;

St. Louis; and the New York area); the Special Needs division of CAJE; a group based at the Minneapolis JCC that does trainings; Familink; West Hennepin Community Service (which will provide inclusion staff to go places with clients); ACT (Acting Change Together); The Tourette's Association; Sha'arim; Lech Lecha; synagogue inclusion committees; selected JFCS programs. (For a complete list, please see the section on Focus Group and Interview Participants' Suggestions in the full report.)

Primary Needs Identified by Respondents

For children, the greatest needs are in the area of inclusive Jewish education (i.e., day school, supplemental school, religious school, Hebrew school). For teens and young adults, the greatest needs are social activities, continuing Jewish involvement, and transportation for both. For adults, the greatest needs are affordable and well-run Jewish housing, social life, and transportation efforts.

ACTIONS AND AGENTS: WHAT YOU CAN DO

(This section can be used as a reference guide to what different parties can do to promote inclusion. There is a list for individuals and families; a list for rabbis, education directors, and other leaders; a list for the Minneapolis Jewish Federation; a list for organizations, including the Minneapolis Jewish Community Center [JCC] and Jewish Family and Children's Services [JFCS], with special sections that apply to synagogues and schools; and a list for the Community Inclusion Program as a whole. This section is intended to take the recommendations from the research—found in the Executive Summary and, in more detail, as summary paragraphs in the Participant Suggestions section [found in the full report]—and make them more concrete and specific. The aim is to help all members of the community move more quickly and effectively to action and, eventually, to full inclusion.)

What Education Directors, Rabbis, and Other Leaders Can Do

- You are the ones called upon to provide moral leadership in inclusion. You need to be the positive role models, the ones who reach out first, and the ones who ensure that an inclusion program is in place in your synagogue or organization, leaders who exemplify and drive inclusion from its basis in Jewish values.

- Question your own values and find ways that you can help people at your synagogue (or other organization) examine theirs. The values that respondents mention–manut (compassion), *Chesed* (loving kindness/loyalty–how one treats others), *Ahavat Yisrael* (love of fellow people/Jews), and *Tikun Olam* (repairing the world)–all have their place in inclusion.
- Deliver a sermon periodically on inclusion and the Jewish values it represents. Give practical suggestions to people so they know what they, as individuals and as a community, can do. Keep the issue alive with your congregation.
- Be open and welcoming to families with a member who has disabilities. Be positive. Show people that their presence is truly desired, not just tolerated.
- Look at your organization's programs and committees and ask yourself, "Are we inclusive? If not, are there things we can do to make it so? Do people with disabilities have representation here?" If not, take action, possibly in concert with the Inclusion Committee.
- Work with your organization's inclusion committee. Show them that you are responsive through your actions. If there is no inclusion committee at your synagogue, lead the drive to find a few core people who will create one.
- Become informed! Read, ask questions, take courses, ask for your organization to carry out trainings and then take part in them yourself. What you learn will be useful to you, your congregation, and to the process of inclusion.
- Help others become informed. Make sure that all staff members in particular have training and knowledge about disabilities. Inquire whether activities and programs are inclusive; get other people to think about what inclusion means. It will make a difference when the questions and suggestions come from you.
- Help publicize disability issues in your synagogue.
- Imagine you are in a wheelchair. Could you get up the curb, in the door, into bathrooms, around all public areas, and onto the *bimah*? If not, let someone know. Again, the fact that you are a rabbi or leader will help your comments about accessibility have greater effect.
- Review the implicit and explicit messages about inclusion taught in your religious school.
- Discourage divisiveness and discrimination in your organization in every form. Have people had disability awareness education?

Are programs inclusive? What are people's understandings of other religions, ethnicities, sexualities, and cultures? Is respect encouraged as an important trait? Are people divided, directly or indirectly, by ability, sexual preference, financial status (as in donation-ranking), level of observance, or in other ways? Does your organization reach out to people through programming and service?

- Invite a person with a developmental disability into your home once a week, once a month, or even once a year. It makes a difference.
- Make sure that there is money set aside for inclusion. It is expensive but vital to the mission of a faith community. Giving scholarships or using a sliding scale for dues or fees is expensive, too, but you do it so that everyone can take part, regardless of income. The same should go for ability. Let your organization's actions reflect the belief that every Jew is deserving of a Jewish education, support from and participation in Jewish institutions, and a role in community life.
- Create opportunities for people with disabilities to teach, lead, serve, work in, and be part of the community.
- Organize or work with a committee at your synagogue or other Jewish organization that can recruit and train volunteers to do child care, welcome people at services or activities, be companions to people with disabilities, visit people in the hospital, tutor children with special needs for B'nai Mitzvah, or make inclusion possible in other ways.
- Support all young people to become B'nai Mitzvah and to become confirmed.
- Meet directly with individuals with disabilities and their families.
- Develop a solid process for working with children with disabilities and their families so that the children can be included and taught well in your religious school programs.
- If someone with a disability (or a family member) comes to you for advice and you don't know who they should talk to or where they should go, find out. Get back to them directly with information or, with their permission, have the appropriate person contact them. Follow up with him/her later to make sure the questions were answered.
- Make arrangements so that ASL signers and/or real-time captioning are available at services when requested.

- Help make transportation possible for members of your congregation or agency. Share in the costs of a wheelchair-accessible bus or van for several organizations. Support fundraising to pay for taxis so that the elderly and other people who cannot drive can attend services and events. Support a ride-share program for the same purpose.
- Keep in mind the needs of teens and adults for social, educational, spiritual, and recreational activities. There tend to be many more inclusive programs for children and many fewer people to advocate on behalf of adults.
- Gauge interest in starting a support or learning group for adults with disabilities, for teens with disabilities, or for family members of people with disabilities. Ensure that those who are affected by "hidden disabilities," including mental illness and learning disabilities, have a place to turn.
- Work with, support, and make use of the Community Inclusion Coordinator's Office.
- Perform outreach and support for unaffiliated Jews, including support groups at organizations such as Courage Center where numerous Christian groups meet.

What the Minneapolis Jewish Federation Can Do

- Make inclusion a funding priority. Show (through funding) that inclusion of people with disabilities is as important as inclusion of other people (such as new immigrants or interfaith families).
- Recognize that while inclusion of people with disabilities may be costly, most programs and other types of inclusion are costly, too. Instead of always separating out what people with disabilities are costing, look at total program costs for each program in terms of what it costs to serve everyone. The Jewish community belongs equally to people with disabilities. Including people with disabilities and their families will certainly help them. It will enrich and vitalize our community just as much. The gains can be tremendous.
- Just as other sorts of diversity and inclusion (such as inclusion of women in decision-making positions or girls in education) should not be limited to a few side programs, inclusion of people with disabilities should be a condition of all organizations and programs in the Jewish community. As the major funder of Jewish organizations, the Minneapolis Jewish Federation has the power to make

inclusion of people with disabilities a condition of funding, just as other organizations, such as the United Way, make non-discrimination a condition of their funding. Setting guidelines now that ask all programs and organizations to become inclusive over the next few years is a powerful form of leadership that the Minneapolis Jewish Federation can exercise.

- Continue to play an important part in building an inclusion program with momentum, substantial impact, and sustainability.
- Consider people with disabilities a target population for the Department of Identity and Continuity at the Minneapolis Jewish Federation. The need here is very great. Many people with disabilities and their families who were not served well or welcomed by the Jewish community have become disenfranchised. Others are on the verge of becoming so. Still others are out in the population of unaffiliated Jews or interfaith families but need the additional draw of knowing that the community is inclusive and welcoming of people with disabilities.
- Make sure that people with disabilities and their families are represented on Federation committees, including those with financial decision-making power.
- Make sure that stakeholders in inclusion–people with disabilities and their families–have the responsibility and the opportunity to be decision-makers, starting now, in terms of priority-setting and allocations.
- Support the central Inclusion Office so that it can take root from the current seed community and continue to grow and thrive within the Minneapolis Jewish community.
- Assist organizations in becoming inclusive. Some possible examples: give incentive grants for specific types of inclusion efforts (such as physical accessibility changes); fund Sha'arim to expand to serve all the children in the community who need their services; provide money to purchase a bus or van with a lift to be shared by community organizations, provided that they maintain the vehicle, hire a driver, and work out logistics for sharing the resource; partner with one or more other organizations to support the development of an office to train trainers who can, in turn, train staff at Jewish institutions.
- Recognize and spread the Jewish values (respondents point to) of *Ahavat Yisrael* (love of fellow Jews), *Chesed* (loving kindness/ loyalty), *Rachmanut* (compassion), and *Tikun Olam* (repairing the world) by promoting inclusion.

- Priorities: For children, the greatest needs are in the area of inclusive Jewish education. For teens and young adults, the greatest needs are social activities, continuing Jewish involvement, and transportation for both. For adults, the greatest needs are affordable, well-run Jewish housing, social life, and transportation.

What Each Program or Organization (Including the JCC and JFCS) Can Do

- Welcome families with a member who has a disability. Be positive. Show people that their presence is truly desired, not just tolerated.
- Take part in building a long-term inclusion program with momentum, substantive changes, positive feeling, and real action.
- Inquire of your organization's programs, "Are they inclusive?" If not, are there things we can do to make them so? Do people with disabilities have representation here? If not, take action, possibly by asking for volunteers from your synagogue's inclusion committee.
- Work with your organization's inclusion committee. Show them that you are responsive through your actions. If there is no inclusion committee at your organization, support the creation of one.
- Make sure that all staff members in particular have training and knowledge about disabilities. It is crucial that leaders, education and program directors, teachers, and counselors are well-trained– and receive continuing education–in disability- and inclusion-related issues. It is also important that other first-contact staff, such as administrative assistants, receptionists, and custodians, are trained so that they can respond appropriately to inquiries and situations that may arise.
- Help publicize disability issues in your organization or synagogue. Ask the editor of the organization's notes, newsletter, or newspaper to include regular updates on inclusion, lists of inclusive programs, and resources for people with disabilities and their families.
- Make your building physically accessible to all.
- Discourage divisiveness and discrimination in your organization in every form. Have people had disability awareness education? Are programs inclusive? What are people's understandings of other religions, ethnicities, and cultures? Is respect encouraged as an important trait? Are people divided, directly or indirectly, by

ability, sexual preference, financial status (as in donation-ranking), level of observance, or in other ways?

- Allocate funds for inclusion. Let your organization's actions reflect the belief that every Jew is deserving of a Jewish education, support from and participation in Jewish institutions, and a role in community life.
- Create opportunities for people with disabilities to teach, lead, serve, work in, and be part of your organization and the community as a whole.
- Make arrangements so that ASL signers and/or real-time captioning are available at services or meetings when requested.
- Help make transportation possible for members of your organization. Share in the costs, maintenance, and logistical facilitation of having a wheelchair-accessible bus or van to meet the community's needs. Alternatively or in addition, support fundraising to pay for taxis so that the elderly and other people who cannot drive can attend work, meetings, events, or services. Support a ride-share program for the same purposes.
- Work with, support, and make use of the Community Inclusion Coordinator's Office.
- Perform outreach that includes Jews with disabilities and their families.
- Reach out to families and individuals with special needs. The initiative should come from within the organization.
- Network about inclusion with other Jewish and non-Jewish organizations, local and national.
- Be inclusive at every age in educational, social, and recreational programs. Give everyone in the community exposure to people with disabilities from a young age so that they are better able to be comfortable, sensitive, and prepared for what may lie ahead in their own futures.
- Counteract staff turnover through thoughtful decision-making, well-supported hires, thorough training, good communication, proactive employee reviews and relations, and clear expectations and goals. People with disabilities and their families invest tremendous time, trust, and energy–all of which may already be overtaxed–in getting to know an inclusion coordinator or education director and developing a relationship with her/him. Their investment is lost, or largely lost, even when there is good record-keeping, if they lose the particular contact. One person is not just as good as another. Since some turnover will still be inevitable, good

record-keeping, close contact with the Community Inclusion Co-ordinator's office, yearly staff training, and good communication can help bridge some of the void until a new person is in place.

- Educate people at all levels and all ages about disabilities, about Jewish values that support inclusion and, in some cases, about Judaism. At least two kinds of education are needed: (1) education and awareness-raising within Jewish organizations about disability issues and inclusion, and (2) education of people in non-Jewish organizations (such as group homes, schools, secular and Christian community resources for people with disabilities) about Judaism, the local Jewish community, and resources within the community. The goals of broad education efforts should include: increasing public awareness; sensitizing people to those who are different; discouraging teasing and mean-spiritedness among children and adults; showing that people with disabilities can be important in their communities; making people with and without disabilities more familiar and comfortable with each other; teaching community members about common disabilities; educating people in the larger community about Judaism and the Jewish community, so that they can serve Jewish clients and members better and refer Jews to services within the Jewish community; welcoming Jews with disabilities and their families back into the Jewish community; providing peer training; empowering people with disabilities; helping people notice and value individuals and focus on what they *are* able to do.

Additionally, for Synagogues

- Gauge interest in starting a support or learning group for adults with disabilities, for teens with disabilities, or for family members of people with disabilities. Ensure that those who are affected by "hidden disabilities," including mental illness and learning disabilities, have a place to turn.
- Review the implications of what is taught in your religious school and what members of your congregation value. Consider addressing inclusion and the value of people in a sermon.
- Organize or work with a committee at your synagogue that can recruit and train volunteers to do child care, welcome people at services or activities, be companions of people with disabilities, visit people in the hospital, tutor children with special needs for B'nai Mitzvah, or make inclusion possible in other ways.

- Support all young people so that they can become B'nai Mitzvah and confirmed.
- Have the appropriate staff person(s) meet directly with individuals with disabilities and their families.
- Develop a solid process for working with children with disabilities and their families so that the children can be included and taught well in your religious school programs.
- If someone with a disability (or a family member of someone with a disability) comes to a staff member for advice and the staff member does not know who the individual should talk to or where s/he should go, that staff person should find out. Get back to the congregant directly with information or, with her/his permission, have the appropriate person make contact. Follow up with question-asker later to make sure her/his questions were answered and her/his needs met.

Additionally, for Schools

- Create Individual Education Plans (IEPs) for and with students.
- Pay special attention to good communication and support with and for students and their parents.
- Create a good process for needs assessment and educational planning.
- Provide extra training on disabilities and inclusion to all teachers.
- Be sure that aids are used in a way that does not isolate a student with a disability more.
- Create or work with an established body (such as Sha'arim) of highly trained professionals and volunteers focused on the education and tutoring of students.
- Make inclusive values, behaviors, and practices a regular part of all students' education.

What the Community Inclusion Office Can Do

- Build a long-term inclusion program with momentum, substantive changes, positive feeling, and real action.
- Make sure that people with disabilities and their families are represented on committees and have the responsibility and the opportunity to be decision-makers, starting now, in terms of priority-setting, allocations, and other issues related to the inclusion program.

- Organize, staff, and support a central Inclusion Office. The existing Inclusion Coordinator position is the perfect beginning, though there may need to be more than one inclusion coordinator and though other resources (such as databases, reading lists, and newsletters) will need to be compiled by the coordinator(s) or by others. Staff in that office can: compile and share information, keep the community focused on true inclusion, assist with communication, link and support organizations and individuals, arrange events and activities, advise committees, advocate on behalf of people with disabilities, help raise money, and be a first-call-for-help and referrals related to disability.
- More specifically, the Community Inclusion Coordinator's Office could serve the community in the following ways:
  - Be a first-call-for-help and community information.
  - See people personally to find out how to serve them.
  - Work with Jewish community organizations to make them more inclusive.
  - Arrange and organize trainings and, possibly, set up a train-the-trainers program, advocate-training, volunteer training, and/or speaker's bureau.
  - Network with other resources and agencies, Jewish and non-Jewish, locally, nationally, and internationally.
  - Be a central clearinghouse of information.
  - Be an advocate for people with disabilities, individually and collectively.
  - Inform religious schools about special education law, presentation of certain curriculum, and best ways to teach a child with a particular disability.
  - Provide information on housing options (including Jewish nursing homes, group homes, independent living buildings, and other arrangements) and transportation possibilities to those who are interested.
  - Bring together and make clearly available information on the special funds for people with disabilities. Assist people in applying for those funds, when appropriate.
  - Let people know what is out there; publicize events, groups, activities, and services.
  - Organize events.
  - Help raise money for inclusion.
  - Lead community inclusion efforts.
  - Help fund-raise in the area of disability.

- Put out a newsletter centered on inclusion.
- Listen to people.
- Run a website with information that may include: Jewish community organizations and synagogues and their status on accessibility and inclusion; Jewish therapists; information on different disabilities; inclusion information on local and national resources; information on other Jewish communities in the USA and internationally; definitions of disability, special needs, and inclusion; numbers to call; lists of books, both fiction and non-fiction, in which characters with disability are central; chat boards.

• Create a centralized resource (within the Community Inclusion Office) which contains information about individuals with disabilities who choose to participate so that they or their parents do not have to repeat everything about themselves and their disability each time they want to take part in a class, program, or activity or each time there is staff turnover. Models could include IEPs and Hennepin County's new seamless K-12 program for children with special needs. The idea behind the centralized file would be that–with a person's consent and control over what is in the file–staff at any Jewish school, camp program, youth group, or other program could become informed efficiently and completely about the person's disability in general, the individual's own personal history, and his/her interests (such as playmates with the same disability or a group home). The result would be that program staff know more and know it faster so that they can be better prepared to work with the individual while the person her/his self (and the person's family) will be freed of hours of repeating themselves. Organizations could continue their inclusion efforts more effectively, even in times of staff turnover.

• Publicize resources effectively. Let people know what exists and how to become involved and included. People need to know about programs before they can take part in them. Information (about resources and inclusion in the Jewish community) needs to be out there in the secular community, too, because that's where many Jews go for support. Advertise over and over until things are read. And be able to respond when people call, which means having receptionists and front-entry people who know about programs and how to relate respectfully.

• Educate people at all levels and all ages about disabilities, about Jewish values that support inclusion and, in some cases, about Judaism. At least two kinds of education are needed: (1) education and awareness-raising within Jewish organizations about disability issues and inclusion, and (2) education of people in non-Jewish organizations (such as group homes, schools, secular and Christian community resources for people with disabilities) about Judaism, the local Jewish community, and resources within the community. The goals of broad education efforts should include: increasing public awareness; sensitizing people to those who are different; discouraging teasing and mean-spiritedness among children and adults; showing that people with disabilities can be important in their communities; making people with and without disabilities more familiar and comfortable with each other; teaching community members about common disabilities; educating people in the larger community about Judaism and the Jewish community, so that they can serve Jewish clients and members better and refer Jews to services within the Jewish community; welcoming Jews with disabilities and their families back into the Jewish community; providing peer training; empowering people with disabilities; helping people notice and value individuals and focus on what they *are* able to do.

What You or Your Family Can Do

- When you serve on a committee or organize a program, think: "Is this program inclusive? Are there things we can do to make it so?" Also, look around you at the composition of the committee. Is it inclusive? Do people with disabilities have representation here? If not, speak up.
- Whether or not you feel informed about inclusion, you can raise the subject at your synagogue, program, or organization. Make sure that staff members in particular have training and knowledge about disabilities. Inquire whether activities and programs are inclusive; get other people to think about what inclusion means.
- If you contribute to a newsletter or newspaper in the Jewish community or the wider community, suggest that the paper regularly cover disability or inclusion issues.
- Become informed! Read, ask questions, take courses, ask for your organization to carry out trainings and then take part in them yourself. What you learn could be useful to you, to others, and to the process of inclusion.

- Ask the Jewish organizations you are part of and the businesses you frequent if they are accessible. Imagine you are in a wheelchair. Could you get up the curb, in the door, into bathrooms, and to all public areas? If not, let someone know.
- Question your values: It is okay to recognize discomfort and uncertainty when interacting with people with disabilities. The question is "What will you do about it?" Some things you can do are to: get more exposure, obtain more knowledge, and/or recognize the differences, abilities, and lacks of ability that everyone (not just those labeled as having a disability) has. Examine your values related to inclusion in general. Are you accepting of others? Do you look down on those with less money, prestige, education, or talent than you? If you have children, what messages do you think you give to them through what you say, what you don't say, what embarrasses you, how you judge people, who you know, what you praise your children for, and how you react to those who are different from you.
- Volunteer. There is a need for advocates, tutors, and support people. Ask for training if it is not already provided.
- Invite a person with a developmental disability into your home once a week, once a month, or even once a year. It makes a difference.
- Offer to drive someone with a disability to services, religious school, or events. If you don't step forward, that person may not be able to attend. If you don't step forward, driving to that same event you are driving to may be another thing for an overburdened parent to do on a long day.
- Volunteer to be a big brother or big sister specifically for a Jewish child with a disability. There are wonderful children who have been waiting for years and are eager to share experiences with adults.
- Volunteer to be a companion to someone your age (a child, teen, or adult) for Jewish activities, services, or classes. You can make the difference on whether that person feels comfortable attending and being a part of the Jewish community or not.
- Offer to baby-sit for a family with a special needs child, even once a month, so the parents can spend time together.
- Offer to be part of a child-care team during services, even once a month, so that parents of children with special needs can attend services.

- Organize or work with a committee at your synagogue or Jewish organization that can recruit and train volunteers to do child care, welcome people at services or activities, be companions of people with disabilities, visit people in the hospital, tutor children with special needs for B'nai Mitzvah, or make inclusion possible in other ways.

CONCLUDING NOTE
FROM THE RESEARCH ADVISORY COMMITTEE

This report marks an important step in the Minneapolis Jewish community's efforts to ensure that everyone can fully participate in all aspects of Jewish life. The recommendations from this report will be prioritized by the community-wide Inclusion Program Steering Committee, which is under the auspices of Jewish Family and Children's Service. Periodic updates measuring the progress of the implementation of these recommendations will be available at a later date. For more information, contact the Community Inclusion Office at 952-542-4838.

NOTES

1. For the purposes of this research, "inclusion" is defined as the opportunity for people with and without disabilities to participate together in educational, spiritual, social, cultural, and recreational activities in the Jewish community.

2. "Disability" is defined as an impairment that limits a person's physical, hearing, vision, communication, social/emotional, developmental, or cognitive function, or impacts a person's learning.

3. Sha'arim is a local independent educational organization that provides special needs Jewish education programs and services on a community-wide basis.

4. Lech Lecha is an ongoing monthly discussion/support group for parents raising a child with special needs administered by Jewish Family and Children's Services.

doi: 10.1300/J095v10n03_10

What Does Being Jewish Mean to You?
The Spiritual Needs of Jewish People
with Learning Disabilities
and Their Families

Eve Kuhr Hersov, EdM, Cert. Gerontology

SUMMARY. This study explores the importance of spiritual, religious, and cultural life among a sample of Jewish people with learning disabilities and their families within Greater London. Emphasis was placed on generating practical ideas and recommendations for improving opportunities for spiritual life and development, plus religious and cultural inclusion. Findings were then reviewed with professionals from Jewish support organisations to better identify and discuss service gaps, needs, and next steps. doi:10.1300/J095v10n03_11 *[Article copies available for a fee from The Haworth Document Delivery Service: 1-800-HAWORTH. E-mail address: <docdelivery@haworthpress.com> Website: <http://www.HaworthPress.com>]*

Eve Kuhr Hersov, is an independent consultant, based in Great Britain, focussing on quality of life issues for people with complex needs. She can be contacted at 23 Willoughby Road, Hampstead, London NW3 1RT England (E-mail: evehersov@msn.com).

This study was commissioned by The Judith Trust, 5 Carriage House, 90 Randolph Ave, London W9 1BG <www.judithtrust.org.uk>, which has given permission for its publication.

[Haworth co-indexing entry note]: "What Does Being Jewish Mean to You? The Spiritual Needs of Jewish People with Learning Disabilities and Their Families." Hersov, Eve Kuhr. Co-published simultaneously in *Journal of Religion, Disability & Health* (The Haworth Pastoral Press, an imprint of The Haworth Press, Inc.) Vol. 10, No. 3/4, 2006, pp. 183-205; and: *Jewish Perspectives on Theology and the Human Experience of Disability* (ed: Rabbi Judith Z. Abrams and William C. Gaventa) The Haworth Pastoral Press, an imprint of The Haworth Press, Inc., 2006, pp. 183-205. Single or multiple copies of this article are available for a fee from The Haworth Document Delivery Service [1-800-HAWORTH, 9:00 a.m. - 5:00 p.m. (EST). E-mail address: docdelivery@haworthpress.com].

Available online at http://jrdh.haworthpress.com

KEYWORDS. Judaism, learning disability, cultural inclusion, identity, London

INTRODUCTION AND AIMS

In the autumn of 2003 The Judith Trust commissioned a piece of research exploring the importance of spiritual, religious, and/or cultural life for Jewish people with learning disabilities and their families. The aim was to survey (in Greater London) a small sample of adults with learning disabilities and parents of people with learning disabilities on the subject, and to generate practical ideas and recommendations for improving opportunities for spiritual life and development, and/or religious and cultural inclusion. As well, it was hoped that service and policy issues would be identified that could then be reviewed and discussed with Jewish social service professionals and community leaders.

GETTING STARTED

Review of Literature and Networking in the Jewish Community

The work commenced examining information and resources concerned with spirituality and learning disability, and contact was made with Dr. John Swinton from the University of Edinburgh and with Dr. Chris Hatton, University of Lancaster, both of whom have completed work on the subject. Concurrent to reviewing literature, efforts also focussed on networking within the Jewish community and identifying potential research participants.

Contact with Adults with Learning Disabilities

Following a meeting with Michael Levin, Norwood's Cultural Advisor (Norwood provides care and support to people with learning disabilities and their families), arrangements were made for the researcher to spend a day at Ravenswood Village (a Jewish residential community for people with learning disabilities run by Norwood) to meet with an established residents group and also with individual residents to discuss the importance of religion, spirituality and culture in their lives. Drawing on the work of John Swinton and Chris Hatton, set questions were devised for the interview and discussion process. Six residents of mixed gender and age participated in the group meeting, three of whom utilised facilitated communication. The group was supported by their regular group leader. Individual interviews were also conducted by the researcher with two residents: a woman in her 30s who lives more independently in a flat at the Village and a man in his 50s who lives in a group home.

The researcher next wanted to interview adults with learning disabilities living in North London. Dawn Preston, Norwood's Adult Opportunities Manager, agreed to circulate a flier advertising a meeting to discuss "What Does Being Jewish Mean to You?" Seven adults with learning disabilities attended the meeting, again comprised of both men and women of a broad age range (20s-70s). The researcher was also able to speak with two middle-aged female members of the group after the meeting to followup several points.

Additionally, the researcher was interested in speaking to adults with learning disabilities who were not living in Jewish group homes or participating in day or leisure services for Jewish adults with learning disabilities. Barnet MENCAP circulated a flier which resulted in two separate individual interviews: a young man in his 20s living at home with parents and a man in his 50s living in a non-Jewish group home.

Contact with Parents

The researcher contacted the Over and Under Fives Support Group (a self-run support group of Jewish North London parents) and information about the research was disseminated. Parents were invited to get in touch with the researcher and eventually an evening meeting was organised comprised of four mothers from the Over and Under Fives Support Group, one father, plus a mother who had heard about the meeting through another parent. A phone interview was conducted with an additional mother who was unable to attend the meeting. All seven of these parents had school-age children.

A second focus group took place with seven mothers from Norwood's Rainbow Group, a support group for Jewish mothers of young children with learning disabilities. Following these two meetings the researcher produced a summary of the comments made by the participating parents which was circulated for response. Interviews were then conducted with a mother from the former Parry (Jewish parents) Group, plus two mothers professionally involved in Jewish organisations that are concerned with learning disabilities. As well, the researcher contacted two fathers who are rabbis.

Contact with Jewish Service Providers and Organisations

The final stage of the research involved networking within the Jewish community. The researcher wanted additional response to the summary of parents comments, particularly in regard to service gaps. But another important aim was to identify resources, examples of good practice, and generate practical suggestions or ideas for further research and/or development. Face-to-face meetings were held with representatives of Norwood, Ezer Northwest (confidential family support), Kisharon (education and care for children and adults with learning disabilities), plus a synagogue Youth Worker, and The Peer Group (synagogue Community Care Coordinators). There was also dialogue with representatives of the Institute for Jewish Policy Research, In Touch (contact group for families with children with special needs), the Community Development Department of the United Synagogue, and the Community Issues Division of the Board of Deputies of British Jews, plus the former head teacher of a Jewish school with experience of integrating special needs children.

FINDINGS–
PARTICIPANTS WITH LEARNING DISABILITIES

The interviews and discussion groups with adults with learning disabilities yielded clear results.

- *Being Jewish was important to people*; **it provided a sense of strength, social belonging and inclusion, and was a part of their personal identity.**

    "My faith keeps me strong when things are difficult for me. It keeps me a part of my family."

    "Being Jewish is my way of life. It makes me who I am."

    "I enjoy being Jewish. It's nice. I love the Jewish holidays we celebrate. I enjoy learning about the Jewish way of life (and traditions); getting married under a chuppah. It means so much to me and it's meaningful. I believe in being a Jewish woman."

- *Judaism offers valued rituals, traditions, and roles* for some people with learning disabilities, such as saying prayers on Shabbat, attending synagogue, and being called to the bimah.

    "I enjoy Shabbat. I enjoy synagogue. I am having a Bat Mitzvah."
    "We have Kiddush Friday nights at the house. I say the prayers."
    "I go to homes to do service."
    "I like being Jewish, eating Jewish food. I like going to shul on Succos, Simchas, Torah, Hanukah and Purim. I don't like going on Rosh Hashanah, Shavuos, and Passover."
    "I been to stone setting." (following the death of a parent)

- *Participation in the celebration of festivals was highly valued.* Singing, dancing, music, and parties were important to people.

    "I love going to Hanukah parties. Each day we get a present and receive Hanukah cards."
    "I like celebrating the festivals."

- *Attending Bar and Bat Mitzvahs and weddings was important* to many participants.

    "I love going to a Jewish wedding."
    "I like Bar Mitzvahs and weddings but I haven't gone for awhile."
    "I go to shul on special occasions; when there is a Bar Mitzvah– a girl or boy is 13, or when a couple get married."

- Religious *observance was seen by many as a sign of respect* for the Jewish faith.

    "I go to the butcher every Friday and it's very important to me to have kosher in my home."
    "He should have more respect for his faith. He's a wally (comments about a resident who attends football on Shabbat.)"

- *Judgement of other peoples' differing degrees of personal observance* clearly exists among some adults with learning disabilities.

    "He's an Arsenal supporter. He usually goes to Highbury. He goes by car. It's got to stop."

"Where I live now we still have loads of arguments about football. I'm entitled (to go). It's my choice."
"I used to go to lunch with the Chazzan (after shul). There was no music. I felt depressed and bored. They were lovely people but I don't approve of being frum."

• **A significant number of** *participants wanted more opportunities for religious and spiritual education* **and development.**

"I'd like lessons about my faith."
"I'd like education in the Torah and history of Judaism."

• **A significant number of** *participants were interested in culture and skill development*; **such as Jewish cooking classes, discussion of Jewish culture and reminiscence.**

"I went to school. I did my Hebrew letters at seven. I'd like to do Jewish cooking."

• **Although the concept of spirituality was generally less easily understood than religion,** *participants* **living in communal setting** *often lacked privacy* **and the personal space necessary for contemplative time.**

"I hate being disturbed when I am trying to sort myself out."
"I (used) to watch the trains go by at Hendon Station British Rail. I don't do it any more (due to staff concerns about safety)."
"I want to be free to travel if I am stressed on a Saturday."

ADDITIONAL COMMENT

There seems much wisdom in Norwood establishing a Cultural Advisor post. Michael Levin's contribution to the organisation was valued by a significant number of the participants (who had an association to Norwood). The role of a Cultural Advisor is important, but the person inhabiting the role is perhaps of greater importance. Michael Levin's enthusiasm for Judaism and his "people" skills and warmth have had a positive impact that goes beyond raising consciousness of Jewishkeit and religion; he adds joy and brings emphasis to essential human traits and values, as well.

INDIVIDUAL INTERVIEWS

It was interesting to note that both men interviewed who had responded to the flier sent out by Barnet MENCAP to adults living in the community (but not associated with Jewish services for people with learning disabilities) had made a conscious choice to seek out a different synagogue.

A

A is a middle-aged man who was raised in an Orthodox family. His parents are no longer alive but he keeps in contact with his remaining sibling and lives in a non-Jewish group home in North London. He talked easily about his life, meeting with the researcher in a Centre for Jewish people.

"I go to synagogue on Saturday. I mix with Jewish and non-Jewish people. I talk to people, go to Bar Mitzvahs and the simchas. I go to my sister every Saturday. She's Jewish–keeps a kosher home."

"It's important (being Jewish). I listen to other people. I get a buzz from being in a Jewish atmosphere. I live in a non-Jewish home and it's OK. I would go to a Jewish home but I think I have enough going to a synagogue. Maybe I should move. I haven't thought about it deeply. I'm settled down. I haven't done too badly."

What's Good About Being Jewish?

"Going to synagogue, talking to Jewish people, identifying with the festivals. I'm learning about the Torah. I mix with people I want to mix with."

"I pray; not as much as I should do. I connect with G-d. It's easier to pray in synagogue. I follow the service."

"I chose my congregation. When I say Haftorah at this synagogue I feel better. The last congregation they didn't call me up but once." (**A** *indicated his present congregation calls him up 2-3 times a year and it is important to him.*) "It's (the new congregation) near where my sister lives. Her congregation is more friendly–men and women sit together–more friendly like." (*Sometimes* **A**'s *sister goes to synagogue with him. Family is clearly important to* **A** *and he spoke about his grown up niece.*)

What's Not So Good About Being Jewish?

"The restrictions. (**A** *has girl friends who aren't Jewish and he feels he cannot take them to synagogue.*) I don't think it matters that my home isn't kosher." (*At this point* **A** *seemed to speak more about what wasn't good in his life, not necessarily related to being Jewish.*) "I'm not marriageable. I'm past the age. Maybe I would have had more chances. . . . (**A**'s *sister indicated in a prior phone call that* **A**'s *mother had been over-protective and that* **A**'s *opportunities expanded following their mother's death.*)

B

B is a man in his early twenties who lives at home with his Orthodox parents. Home life is not ideal and there are tensions. **B** has consciously chosen to attend an Ultra-Orthodox synagogue. **B** was eager to communicate about Judaism.

"I'm very, very Orthodox. Jewish means to me quite a lot. I believe in Judaism. G-d told us to take certain decisions; circumcision, Bar Mitzvah, tefillin, marriage."

"On Shabbos I'd like to make my own Kiddush. At home my father doesn't let me. He does it for me. I don't know why. At other people's houses I make my own."

"It's hard for me to find a wife because I suffer from (**B** *mentions a medical condition*). . . . I can't find a girl friend."

B *changed synagogues* "because I wanted to become more Hassidish–from Ashkenazic to Sephardic." **B** *explained that the Rav invited him home for a Shabbos meal.* "My family don't want me to be Hassidish. I like the way they daven (pray) even though the Rav speaks Yiddish which I don't understand."

B *seems to find people more welcoming at the Hassidic synagogue. He recounted being invited to a congregant's home after attending a Bar Mitzvah whereas at his previous synagogue he wasn't invited back to congregants' homes, even when his parents were invited.*

B *has had no contact with Jewish social service organisations. He did attend a Jewish school for young people with learning disabilities but described it as "restrictive" as he feels they did not respect his religious observance needs adequately.*

"On Saturday I go to a study group at my synagogue and work with a man who teaches a few (younger) boys." **B** *appears frustrated because* *it seems that even though the Hassidic synagogue is more welcoming to him, he still does not easily fit into a peer group.* **B** relates, "There is no one there to team me with."

"I need classes–Hebrew studies." **B** *appears isolated. He speaks about wanting to participate in sports like cricket and football and says*, "It doesn't have to be a Jewish team."

FINDINGS–PARENTS

The two focus groups and parent interviews raised numerous issues.

- **Parents want greater *inclusion* for their children; a way for their learning disabled children to join in synagogue and community life. Parents also want to know about existing good practice.**

  > "I want him to go to Cheder or at least a Jewish group to learn songs and about festivals."
  > "On the High Holidays I used to go to my mother's shul. They had a crèche. But they were not geared up for a special needs child. I gave up trying to take him."
  > "In Leicester, they put a tallis on my son and asked if he would open the ark with his cousin. It was lovely for me."

- **Parents want a *designated person* or people at synagogue whose role is to provide information, support and to facilitate inclusion and instruction for their disabled child.**

  > "The parent of the disabled child could advise the rabbi, teachers, or other mentors on their child's needs, as well as their need for support from the community. Rabbis and synagogues should become informed about people with special needs, and how to meet educational, spiritual, practical and community needs through Jewish and synagogue life."
  > "Who supports the designated person at synagogue? No do-gooders, please! This person must be well-supported, too. Maybe more than one person in case of absence or illness. It is dreadful for a family to arrive expecting support and then be let down yet again."

- **Parents want *Rabbis to get special training* on how to deal with parents of a disabled child and how to better include disabled children into their congregations.**

- **Some parents raised the need for mentoring and *youth programmes*, and also spoke of the value of groups that integrate youngsters.**

> "We started out with Norwood and there was good support but after age 5 it fell off. There is a need for ongoing service. Now that my child is 11, I'd like a Jewish secondary school play group."
>
> "He loves being with children his own age and joins in as he can."
>
> "In a mainstream environment he is encouraged to develop a personality."

- **Parents want access to a variety of *resources*: in regard to disability, the Jewish community, and appropriate easily understood educational tools and materials about Judaism, Bar Mitzvah, Jewish culture, etc.**

> "So many of the books aren't simple enough or textural; music, symbols–they all help."
>
> "The tools and materials could be used within the community or to help the disabled synagogue member to access as much of Jewish and synagogue life as possible."

- **Parents want and need *sensitive and timely support from both local authority professionals and their faith community*. Many parents mentioned that often support is offered by professionals at times when parents are not able to take on the information given. For this reason parents felt it would be useful to have *written resource materials* (like a handbook) available that they could refer back to and a way for this information to be updated.**

> "You have just given birth and don't understand about non means tested benefits like DLA,"
>
> "You don't need respite yet."

- **Mothers currently and formerly involved in the Norwood therapeutic play group (the Rainbow Group) valued this *support group* highly.**

    "It was *the* place. I had people I could talk to. I felt I had joined a club."

    "It was my one and only support."

    "I liked coming. It was the one place I trusted someone to look after my son. I went for my child. I wouldn't have left the house for myself."

    "My husband went (to the father's support group) and loved it."

    "There was a lot of gallows humour (in the Father's Group). It was liberating."

- **Parents emphasized two specific needs: improving the mechanisms for *how information is disseminated* to Jewish parents, and improving the mechanisms for *identifying Jewish parents* who have a learning disabled child.**

    Parents participating in this research who had attended a Norwood support group for mothers (or their group for fathers) indicated that they had often learned about the group by happenstance.

    "Every Jewish person with a disabled child should be told about Norwood. People find out by chance. Norwood needs to send out booklets to every shul, child development centre, and nursery. New synagogue members should get a welcome pack with info on Norwood."

- **Parents want to be able to *access a flexible range of care* and need reassurances about what is available now and in future.**

    Some parents with children at home have fears about accessing care in future. For instance, one parent who did not yet feel the need for respite care, expressed the worry that if she did not get her foot in the door with respite care now, that later when she was older and would need more assistance she wouldn't be able to access it.

- **Religious parents prioritise the need for their children to be educated in a *Jewish school*.**

Parents expressed concern that Kisharon School cannot take children in wheelchairs or with certain diagnoses, and spoke of the reluctance of local authorities to provide funding at Kisharon; leaving many parents with no option but to accept education in a non-Jewish school.

> "There's no provision in the Jewish sector for my children. I'm torn. I can't send them to Cheder. It's my biggest disappointment."
> "It's devastating."
> "There is an EU ruling about the right to education in religious schools but the UK has a clause inserted making this dependent upon resources so we do not have a choice."

- **Some parents expressed interest in the American concept of a** *Jewish Community Centre* **(that is non-affiliated), where the emphasis is on providing** *cultural, spiritual, social and recreational activities* **(not religious activity) to the entire Jewish population.**

> "It is for everyone." Parents readily appreciated that there were Jewish needs to be met outside of religious or synagogue life, for themselves and especially for their families.
> "For families like ours–that don't fit into a shul (because our child cannot cope)–we should be talking about it."

- **Many parents complain of** *intolerance and ignorance* **of disability in regard to synagogue life and within the commercial Jewish community.**

> "I've had more trouble in the local Jewish deli than in M & S. I've been more embarrassed there; they snap at him.
> At synagogue: "It is fear of the unknown; of saying or doing the wrong thing."

INDIVIDUAL INTERVIEWS

Mrs. C

Mrs. C is the mother of a middle-aged child **D**, who lives in a Jewish group home. Mrs. C became involved about 30 years ago in The Parry

Group–Jewish parents who fundraised and campaigned to open the first Jewish group home in London.

"We had a vision and we realized it. We wanted a home before we were no longer here. This is why we started up the group. We had a rabbi–Rev. Gerald Schneider. It was announced at all the synagogues. There was a meeting in one parent's home and it grew–25 families in the Redbridge area. We had somebody to talk to."

Regarding the Group Home Where Her Child Lives

"It's wonderful. They are happy. **D** has a peer group. **D**'s with friends. We have the greatest satisfaction knowing that **D** will be looked after."

"Every 3-4 months we have a parents meeting. We get together and we talk. **D**'s house knows of (another relative) who they can look to (should something happen to me)."

"The staff are younger than **D**. They have energy and they integrate **D** into Jewish activities. **D**'s proud of herself and goes to College. We can't give **D** what the home provides."

Mrs. E

Mrs. E has a pre-teenage son, **F**, living at home.

"For **F**, the connection (in synagogue) is instant. I think it is based on the music. You know where you are. It is a calming effect."

"We've had to go and ask for everything (regarding Local Authority). **F** can't walk or talk. **F** responds differently (better) in a normal environment.

"Now **F** has been invited to attend the Youth Service. He sits next to his father in Shul and attends regularly."

Mrs. G

Mrs. G is professionally involved in learning disability work and has an adult learning disabled child.

"I've been on a very long painful journey."

". . . (Some families) shut down at the point of diagnosis–it's emotionally disabling. There's the pariah thing. You have to survive and function in a practical way. You lose spontaneity as a family. Disability dominates family life."

"Many years ago I attended a half-day seminar. Something said there changed my life and the way I viewed myself and other parents. It was research saying that the way doctors (and others) give the diagnosis/prognosis affects the family for the next 20 years. Eureka! So this is why I had been feeling so angry–the experts had given me no hope . . . This needs to be addressed."

"My interest in spirituality is great. For me it involves connecting in a true, honest and genuine way with other human beings. It means connecting from the heart. It means being with each other because we truly want to share with them."

"Religion can be great, too. It is different (from spirituality). It gives us structure, tradition, and rituals. However, for religion to be meaningful to anyone it needs to meet them where they are and it needs to be presented in ways people can understand and use and that are meaningful to them. No good gabbling on in Hebrew when English is a struggle."

"The most moving and powerful experience I have had was some years ago, the late Cardinal Basil Hume said a prayer to 100's of people including many, many families of people with learning disabilities. The sentence was short and so simple and went something like 'G-d loves me and protects me and is here by my side.' He got everyone to repeat it many times."

Rabbi H

Rabbi H has an adult learning disabled child. He spoke easily about his early experiences and how as a young rabbi he was unprepared and inexperienced in regard to helping families with disabled children, and unable to easily ask for help himself as a father.

"As a young rabbi, I wouldn't have helped me."

"Had I pushed (for support) there would have been rabbis who helped (me)."

Rabbi H spoke about how he eventually received support from Jewish and Local Authority services.

"Rabbi Baum (whose wife set up a toy library) set up a day seminar for rabbis. Only one rabbi knew of our situation and not much (about our child). I went to the seminar and I heard a guest speaker describe families and she described me, and I realized that I was normal. I went to see her and she introduced us to Mrs . . . (from Ravenswood). We actually then got snowed under with help."

Rabbi H and his wife have addressed support groups for Jewish parents. He relates that "people (parents of disabled children) have come to us."

Rabbi H is sensitive to the situation in many Orthodox homes where "Mums raise children" and "Mums can be isolated." He also acknowledges that there can be secrecy about disability in some families and concerns about how disability might affect the future life of other children, especially in regard to making a shiddach (a marriage).

ADDITIONAL COMMENT

Several additional themes emerged during the process of trying to develop focus groups or interviews with parents and during interviews.

- Many *mothers of young children* describe a life that is complicated by *social isolation*. This was voiced by mothers from across the full spectrum of religious observance, but seemed especially poignant amongst some more observant Jews.
- The majority of parents who participated were either young or middle-aged. The researcher had greater difficulty accessing older parents. Some older parents known to the researcher were significantly silent. There was reluctance to being involved in the research. In certain cases it may be that the topic of the research created *discomfort*, in others there may have been discomfort in just looking backwards. There is no doubt that many parents interviewed–across the age spectrum and the range of religious observance–had *difficulty coming to terms emotionally and spiritually with the birth of a disabled child.*
- There exists amongst many Jews a degree of *self-consciousness*, particularly *around religious observance*. There was more success in scheduling one focus group for parents after changing the title of the group meeting to "You don't have to be religious, just Jewish!" The researcher had been told that parents might have been staying away because they feared they would be judged; they may have assumed that the research topic was geared towards "religious" Jews.

FINDINGS–
CONTACT WITH JEWISH SERVICE PROVIDERS
AND ORGANISATIONS

Networking amongst the Jewish community was a varied experience for the researcher. Gaining access or information from individuals and organisations ranged from being extraordinarily easy and direct in many instances, to taking months to develop.

The researcher was often impressed by the enthusiasm with which the research was welcomed, but noted that *linkage between organisations seems underdeveloped.* Dr. Rona Hart, of the Community Issues Division of The Board of Deputies of British Jews, told the researcher that the Jewish community in Britain is "highly networked, but information doesn't flow." This has clear implications as the ability to access information and support is crucial to improving quality of life for people with learning disabilities and their families.

Response from Direct Service Providers (Support Agencies, Synagogue Care Coordinators, Educators, and Rabbis)

The researcher circulated a written summary of issues raised by parents and engaged in dialogue via telephone and face-to-face meetings. Further discussion of the research and findings yielded the following comments and issues.

In Regard to the More Orthodox Community

- "Within the Orthodox community there can be a conflict between parents' desires, what the reality is (regarding the severity of the disability), and the response of religious leaders."
- "*Parents may have unrealistic ideas* about services and (unrealistic) expectations."
- "The *spiritual and emotional issues of parents may not be easily addressed. There are high levels of denial and unresolved grief.*"
- "The perceptions of *parents need to be addressed* (even if they aren't accurate)." *Many mothers perceive that they are rejected within the religious community.*
- "A lot *of women are on their own.* There is an unspoken issue–unsupported wives."
- "*The community is private.*"
- There are key differences between the more Orthodox and the modern or non-Orthodox community. For the more Orthodox, there is a smaller pool of resources to access "because you can't. . . ." Norwood might not be seen as Orthodox enough because they mix genders. "*The girl-boy issue*" is often an unaddressed problem.

But separating the sexes has implications beyond education or residential care. For instance, adolescent girls in the more Orthodox community finish school at 4 p.m. and can volunteer to help learning disabled children, but they cannot work with adolescent or pre-adolescent boys; leaving a significant service gap.

David Goodman, Executive Director of Kisharon, acknowledged the struggles that families face and spoke powerfully about inclusion.

"Every family has had to fight for their (learning disabled) child to have a Jewish education; whereas their non-disabled children have a choice of Jewish schools. And if they managed to get (their disabled child) into a Jewish school—it is a major battle."
"Every child, whether learning disabled or not, has the right to be a welcomed member of the (Jewish) community."

The Peer Group (Synagogue Care Coordinators)

The researcher met with seven members of The Peer Group plus a synagogue youth worker to discuss the research and gain feedback. The members represented five synagogues with a range of affiliation: Reform, Liberal and Progressive, and United Synagogue (Orthodox). In some synagogues the Care Coordinator's role is primarily concerned with ageing members which in one congregation comprised 33% of the membership. In regard to the five congregations represented at the meeting, one Care Coordinator's remit was exclusive to the elderly while another Care Coordinator had never had contact with learning disabled members or their families as no one had ever been in contact. Elsewhere, there has been a more proactive approach.

The Community Support Coordinators from Edgware and District Reform Synagogue have talked to synagogue staff about their work and are looking towards a "whole synagogue approach" regarding complex special needs. They have held meetings and started a support group for parents that placed priority on generating practical ideas about support and resources. Plans include developing one-to-one support for children with complex needs and designing a special needs Bar and Bat Mitzvah programme.

The Peer Group summarized the issues that hold back progress in regard to greater inclusion of people with learning disabilities within synagogue and community life and identified specific needs:

- *"Manpower and money"*–funding is needed to address community needs. "It's budget time in shuls–everyone is struggling."
- *There needs to be an audit* to better identify the population of people with learning disabilities, and to find out their requirements, and what they want.
- *There needs to be leadership* and directives from the Board of Deputies of British Jews. "It has to come *from the top.*"
- *There needs to be better communication, links, and sharing.* The group mentioned the need for better web information and links, as well as improving media coverage from the *Jewish Chronicle* and the *London Jewish News*. There was acknowledgement that "religion can get in the way of sharing (information)." The differences in religious observance and background amongst London Jews can be a barrier to the flow of information. But it was also noted that the internal communication within synagogues was often problematic; that the Education Department might not link with Care Coordination, etc.
- *There needs to be a proactive approach with people and families*–One Care Coordinator expressed, "When I started seven years ago I was fearful of being intrusive and proactive. Now I pick the phone up." She felt that her current concerns were about not having people or families "fall through the cracks."
- *There is still shame*–It was felt in some instances that families of children with special needs still felt a degree of shame which inhibited their asking for help.

Additional Comments and/or Issues Identified by Other Direct Service Providers

- **Pain, shame, and emotional conflict**

    "What came through to me from your findings is the enormous *pain* parents are still feeling."
    "There are *connotations (for mothers) about having more children.* They talk about the implications of having more children and the impact on (their other) children."
    "*It's a generational thing* (some older parents not responding to the research)." "They may not feel capable or they may feel *shame* (regarding older parents not taking a learning disabled child to synagogue)."

"We have one service user who got a call that her father passed away. He was buried and the mother didn't tell her till after. *She was excluded.*"

- **Enormous time pressures/overwhelming tasks faced by parents caring for children with complex special needs.**

"Mothers (of young children) are very focused on statements, education, appointments, different therapies."

Rabbi Dr. Julian Shindler expressed, "There are so many hurdles you have to jump over if you have a child with special needs. You write to this one and that one. Every time you open a letter there's another thing you have to do. . . . Everything is an appointment. . . . You're trying to run a house; you have a job to do . . . "

The researcher spoke to Toby Walzer, of In Touch, about the emotional issues faced by families. Toby Walzer expressed that individual personality plus support play a major part in how parents come to terms with the birth of a disabled child. She said, "We are all for this and we want to achieve this–coming to terms with feelings." In Touch has a membership of 120 Orthodox families throughout England. They hold frequent meetings focused on providing information and help (rabbinical, legal, medical, etc.), publish a magazine, organise a yearly respite trip for mothers, plus have a siblings group–Kids United.

A former head teacher at a Jewish school spoke positively about inclusion, relating, "I worked hard to have the (disabled) children included. I had to work in advance with the teachers. We managed quite well. The (non-disabled) children were marvellous (about accepting disability)."

The head teacher went on to talk about issues in regard to parents, stating, "*Denial (of disability) is big.* I think particularly so in Britain." "Years ago the government sent out a booklet for parents–Parents Choice. It raised huge expectations in parents. It was mean to raise hopes. Ordinary primary schools don't have teachers trained (in regard to serious disability)." "Head teachers can't deliver and that's hard; extraordinarily demoralizing. It often becomes a battlefield of dissatisfied parents who feel their children should make more progress." "*It is humiliating for parents to beg.*" The head teacher concluded that there were also issues around government funding, and *information that "is unwieldy* and demoralizing to work your way through."

Response from Jewish Community Organisations and Individuals

Dr. Rona Hart, of the Community Issues Division of The Board of Deputies of British Jews, is currently involved in developing a handbook for adults with special needs. This follows on an existing (Board of Deputies) publication, "Special Needs–A guide for parents and carers of Jewish children with special educational needs." A sociologist, Dr. Hart related that "*disability affects belonging*" and results in people feeling "less embedded in the community; (they) relate to the community through their shul only." Her own research corroborates concerns voiced by certain parents; that "having a disabled child at home is (seen as) a shame" and, as well, the "lack of tolerance" encountered in shul. The notion of *propriety* within British culture was discussed along with the strong control mechanisms that exist that reinforce this idea of "behaving properly." Dr. Hart also mentioned how social status can be jeopardized by disability.

Dr. Winston Pickett, Director, External Relations at the Institute for Jewish Policy Research, spoke with the researcher about British Jewish consciousness. When meeting with the Rainbow (support) Group (for mothers), it had been noted that a particular mother felt bitter about the lack of support she received from friends within the Jewish community. The researcher asked at that time whether the mother had ever asked her friends for help, and she had not. Dr. Pickett concurred that within British Jewry "*there is reluctance to ask for help.*" Indeed, people may be willing to help but are not proactive. Dr. Pickett mentioned a survey of Jews conducted in London and the Southeast where many people expressed interest in the idea of doing voluntary work but don't then actively seek out opportunities.

In regard to the findings, Dr. Pickett expressed that "*Jewish culture works*"; that the idea as expressed by parents for a Jewish Community Cultural Centre is a positive step that *brings people together*. He stated the importance of highlighting the issues that face people with learning disabilities and their families; and the need to utilize the media, too, in the process of "acknowledging problems" and "getting people together" to move things forward.

CONCLUSION

The adults with learning disabilities who participated in this research study all identified themselves as Jews and seemed to derive positive satisfaction from different aspects of the religion and culture. Being a Jew seemed to provide a sense of belonging. For some participants there was clear pride in their heritage and background, while others focused more on the importance of observance, religious study or the pleasure of communal celebrations. While the concept of spirituality was less well understood, everyone valued having a sense of "connectedness" with other people, and some participants spoke eloquently about G-d, prayer, and the value of having time and a place to reflect. Although it was noted that living in a group home could impact negatively on opportunities for finding peace and quiet.

When conducting the focus groups for adults with learning disabilities, the researcher was impressed by the impassioned views and feelings of the participants. Each group thanked the researcher and indicated that they enjoyed the opportunity to discuss what being Jewish meant to them. Specific participants had clear ideas about how they would like to further develop their religious or Jewish cultural life. But in each instance, these individuals needed support to put this development into action. It appeared that despite each participant having a clear link to the Jewish community, either through receiving a specific service (residential or leisure) or through affiliation with a synagogue, no one was accustomed to being asked about how they would like to further develop their religious or cultural life.

The failure to ask adults with learning disabilities what they want and aspire to in their religious and cultural life highlights a gap in what Jewish organisations and synagogues provide. The gap seems more serious when we consider that many of the participants are not empowered to ask for help and have limitations on their life experience. The onus is on the wider community and service organizations to assist people in developing positive and fulfilling lives; maximising the opportunities for greater participation and involvement in faith and culture.

The parents involved in this research study clearly want greater inclusion in Jewish life for their children. Additionally, parents articulated a sense of frustration in accessing information and resources to assist them in this process. Some mothers of young children spoke about feeling socially isolated and felt that the Jewish community lacked tolerance. There is no doubt that parents can feel overwhelmed by the sheer volume of task and effort involved in caring for a disabled child. In the hierarchy of needs, religion and spiritual life may take lower priority than physical health and education, especially as so many parents are exhausted by the battle to attain appropriate schooling for their children. But inclusion in synagogue and a greater sense of accep-

204 Jewish Perspectives on Theology and the Human Experience of Disability

tance in the Jewish community are both crucial to achieving a better quality of life for people with learning disabilities and their families.

Generally speaking, the needs outlined by parents fall into three broad categories; *inclusion, support, and access to information*. Discussion with direct service providers and Jewish community organisations about the service gaps in these areas helped to clarify issues.

It seems to the researcher that in order to move forward on inclusion, support, and access to information there needs to be *improved communication and linkage between all stakeholders*. These stakeholders include families, people with learning disabilities, Jewish service providers, non-Jewish service providers working with Jewish clients, synagogues, Jewish community organisations, and the Jewish media. Once communication lines are open it becomes easier to address all problems.

For instance, *parents need better information about resources*. They want to know who can help them and where to get materials to further their child's inclusion in Jewish life. They want to know which synagogues have youth clubs for disabled children or where to find a Bar or Bat Mitzvah tutor. At present there is no clear route to this information. Parents have a vested interest in good practice but are often left on their own to find information because even the professionals in the Jewish community are not well linked up to help. Resources and good practice exist but finding out about them is time consuming, adding to the high stress levels already experienced by families.

A third related issue which again ties into improving communication and linkage is the need to establish *protocols about identifying, approaching and supporting Jewish people with learning disabilities, and their parents* and families. Many parents feel under-supported and isolated despite participating in established support groups. Some parents find asking for help difficult. So it can become more problematic if greater help is needed than might already be provided. This can leave parents feeling embarrassed, humiliated, and/or self-conscious about their situation; all feelings that further marginalise families who yearn for normalcy and inclusion in their community.

Parents expressed that they often found support by coincidence. This was disconcerting to them, and again, contributed towards their sense of isolation. Parents wanted clearer entry into relevant Jewish services, and along with professionals expressed concern that families needing help might be overlooked or "fall through the cracks." Setting up protocols for identifying and approaching families would certainly address parents' perceptions of being unsupported, while also improving access to existing services.

NEXT STEPS

There is no doubt that changes are necessary to create a better quality of Jewish life for Jewish people with learning disabilities and their families. How those changes are brought about requires commitment from the Jewish community in regard to time and funding. The way forward is not entirely clear or direct but certain ideas have been expressed during this research and further discussion of them is recommended.

- To engage with the Jewish media to raise consciousness amongst the Jewish community around the issues of inclusion, communication, and support.
- To fund research looking into good practice, especially in regard to inclusion.
- To compile a list of available resources and improve access to this information through print publication and/or via the Internet.
- To organise meetings to address specific issues such as:
  - establishing better communication and linkage between support organisations, synagogues, people with learning disabilities and parents.
  - developing protocols for identifying and approaching people with learning disabilities or their parents. Care Co-ordinators mentioned the idea of synagogues auditing their membership to identify whether they had people with learning disabilities amongst their membership who could benefit from further support and contact.
- To identify "champions" or leaders amongst the Jewish community committed to inclusion, communication, and information sharing who can steer the way towards change.

doi: 10.1300/J095v10n03_11

Marriage and Parenthood Among Persons with Intellectual Disability in Jewish Law

Isack Kandel, MA, PhD
Katherine Bergwerk, MD
Joav Merrick, MD

SUMMARY. This paper examines the attitude of the Jewish Law towards marriage and parenthood in persons with intellectual disability (ID). The criterion for validity of a marriage is a minimal level of understanding (known as daat kpeutot which is equivalent to the level of a six-year normally developed child) and the comprehension of the act of mar-

Isack Kandel is Senior Lecturer at the Faculty of Social Sciences, Department of Behavioral Sciences, the Academic College of Judea and Samaria, Ariel. During the period 1985-93 he served as Director of the Division for Mental Retardation, Ministry of Social Affairs, Jerusalem, Israel (E-mail: kandelii@zahav.net.il).

Katherine Bergwerk formerly of the Cedars-Sinai Medical Center, Los Angeles, where she was Associate Clinical Professor of Ophthalmology, Jules Stein Eye Institute, UCLA, is now working in private practice in Israel (E-mail: Bergwerk@juno.com).

Joav Merrick is the Director of the National Institute of Child Health and Human Development, Division of Pediatrics, Faculty of Health Sciences, Ben Gurion University, Beer-Sheva and also Medical Director at the Division for Mental Retardation, Ministry of Social Affairs, Jerusalem, Israel (E-mail: jmerrick@internet-zahav. net).

[Haworth co-indexing entry note]: "Marriage and Parenthood Among Persons with Intellectual Disability in Jewish Law." Kandel, Isack, Katherine Bergwerk, and Joav Merrick. Co-published simultaneously in *Journal of Religion, Disability & Health* (The Haworth Pastoral Press, an imprint of The Haworth Press, Inc.) Vol. 10, No. 3/4, 2006, pp. 207-216; and: *Jewish Perspectives on Theology and the Human Experience of Disability* (ed: Rabbi Judith Z. Abrams and William C. Gaventa) The Haworth Pastoral Press, an imprint of The Haworth Press, Inc., 2006, pp. 207-216. Single or multiple copies of this article are available for a fee from The Haworth Document Delivery Service [1-800-HAWORTH, 9:00 a.m. - 5:00 p.m. (EST). E-mail address: docdelivery@haworthpress.com].

riage. Jewish Law maintains that if the person understood the meaning of being married, even if the person did not intend the ceremonial act of marriage, the act itself would be considered valid. This attitude is much more understanding and liberal in comparison to American Law, which has forbidden such marriages. A case anecdote is presented and the implications for child development growing up as a child of a parent with intellectual disability are discussed. There is a paucity of information on the number of such cases, and only sparse information on the effects on these children. However, one recent study demonstrated a contrasting picture of resilience and a close warm relationship by these children later on in life with their family and especially their mother. doi:10.1300/J095v10n03_12 *[Article copies available for a fee from The Haworth Document Delivery Service: 1-800-HAWORTH. E-mail address: <docdelivery@haworthpress.com> Website: <http://www.HaworthPress.com>* © 2006 by The Haworth Press, Inc. All rights reserved.]

KEYWORDS. Intellectual disability, developmental disability, mental retardation, parents with intellectual disability, Jewish Law, Israel

In the modern State of Israel marriage is an act based on religious law or Halacha, and the rabbinate is the only established authority that is sanctioned to perform a marriage ceremony. This paper will discuss the attitude of the Jewish Law towards marriage and parenthood in persons with intellectual disability (ID).

THE CONCEPT OF MARRIAGE IN JUDAISM

In Judaism, marriage is the ideal human state of affairs and considered the basic institution established by G-d from the time of creation. In the Bible it is clearly stated that the purposes of marriage are companionship and creation of the next generation with the following statement for companion: "It is not good that man should be alone, I will make him a help for him. . . . Therefore shall a man leave his father and his mother and shall cleave into his wife and they shall be one flesh" (Gen. 2:18, 24) and the other for creation: "Be fruitful and multiply and replenish the earth. . . ." (Gen. 1:28).

The marriage ceremony described in the Bible is referred to as simply "taking a wife" (Deut. 24:1), but from several cases (Jacob, Leah and

Rachel) it can be understood that there were socially defined rules and customs. In the Talmud (the oral law) the marriage ceremony has two parts. The first, kiddushin or erusin (betrothal), *took* place when the bridegroom gave any object of value (a ring, for example) to the bride and said in front of two witnesses: "With this ring you are consecrated to me according to the law of Moshe and Israel." The second stage took place at a later date (up to a year later) with the marriage proper or nisuin or the Chuppah and was effected after the bride is brought to the house of the groom and cohabited with him. Today in modern Israel both the kiddushin and the Chuppah take place at the same event, usually in a wedding hall with the families from both sides and their friends. Different ethnic groups (like Sephardim or Yemenite Jews) have variations with different traditions.

LEGAL ASPECTS OF MARRIAGE

According to the religious Jewish Law, every man can marry following his a "bar mitzvah" (ceremony at the age of 13 years) after which he is qualified and obligated to fulfill all the religious laws. From 0-13 years he is called a minor (katan) without any legal status, but by 13 years he is called a gadol (an adult). A female is a minor until the age of 12 years, a "naarah" (an adolescent) until 12-and-a-half years and only afterwards an adult. From 12 to 12-and-a-half she will have to have the permission of her father to marry, but afterwards she is considered an adult.

Child marriage as such in Jewish Law is not a problem as long as the male is 13 years and the female 12-and-a-half years old, but in modern Israel the law has been amended and a female cannot marry before the age of 17 years of age. The male, who marries a female under 17 years of age, will be punished by imprisonment, a fine or both. However district courts have jurisdiction to permit a marriage to a girl under 17 years, when she has had a child or is pregnant by the male, or if there are other special circumstances which permit the marriage, provided the girl is not under 16 years of age. Today this is very rare in Israel, while in the past with the immigration from Yemen or North Africa several cases took place.

The criterion for validity of a marriage is a minimal level of understanding (called daat kpeutot or the intellectual capacity of a six-year normally developed child) and the comprehension of the act of marriage

(Merrick et al., 2001). The status of a person with intellectual disability in Jewish Law is complicated due to a lack of a definition both in the Bible and the Talmud (Lifshitz & Merrick, 2001). The Halacha differentiates between people who have developed normally and those defined as deranged or deaf or shotah, with a mental capacity disorder and thought process or behavioral process impaired (Lifshitz & Merrick, 2001). The deranged can suffer from mental illness, melancholy, brain injury or diseases of old age or any other reason, but the Halacha does not make a difference between them and does not categorize them according to etiology, but rather according to level of functioning. Deafness was in the same category as deranged, because communication was compromised.

Halacha recognizes situations in which a person functions at a level lower than "daat kpeutot," but is nevertheless capable of understanding the significance of the act of marriage. This possibility was described by Rabbi Raphael Lipman Halperin (the "Oneg YomTov," Poland, 19th century) and cited by Farbstein (1995):

> . . . a man with a speech defect making his words extremely difficult to understand, and even people used to his company do not always understand his speech, and his mind is very weak, and does not even know how to count, he does not understand the meaning of divorce at all, and it never occurred to him to divorce, because never, since his birth, has he known that divorce exists in the world, and he does not even know anything about the Torah. And whatever he does, he does only because he has habitually seen others doing these things . . .
>
> This man's acts of marriage are valid acts, because we have seen that he can adopt acts that he regularly sees in his environment; this person has the legal status of one who is intelligent, because when something is explained, it makes sense to him.

In other words, the Rabbis take into account situations where people with ID may exhibit greater and lesser abilities in different areas of functioning, being very deficient in one domain, while being able to understand complex actions in another. Therefore, Rabbi Halperin maintained that if the person understood the meaning of being married, even if the person did not understand the ceremonial act of marriage, the act itself would be considered valid. This position has become Halacha or law.

CHILDREN

Once a Jewish man has passed "bar mitzvah" he is obliged to fulfill the command "be fruitful and multiply," but as mentioned above today in modern society males wait a little longer in order to get married and multiply. In order to fulfill this commandment, a male and a female child have to be born, so even after seven girls the commandment has not been fulfilled.

So for a couple, where one or both are persons with ID, there are no restrictions on having children according to Jewish Law. Sterilization is another complicated matter, where Jewish Law is against sterilization of men, but this does not apply to women (Jakobovits, 1959).

A CASE STORY

The family in question lived in a religious neighborhood in Jerusalem. The father, age 40 years, was born in Israel, functions marginally, and did not work. Instead he spent his time studying in a Yeshiva (study hall). The mother, 37, was born in the United States, and immigrated to Israel at the age of 14 years. As a child in the United States she was removed from her home by a court order and adopted. She mainly grew up in a boarding school and entered in to an arranged marriage at the age of 18. This religious family, of Ashkenazi origin, with both parents exhibiting borderline to mild intellectual disability, has 11 children.

The wife is able to read, write a little and able to fill out forms, combined with an amazing ability of speech. She speaks continually, illogically, and without limits. Her parenting abilities are minimal, as evidenced in the children, who have reached the danger point as far as their health and mental welfare is concerned. There is emotional and environmental deprivation.

The father spends all the time in the Yeshiva, with very minimal, if any, time in the house. He leaves the house by 6:30AM and arrives home by 22:00 PM every day. The social worker maintains that the husband is "insignificant" at home, as father and husband. Social Services have known the family, since the birth of the children, due to the level of neglect and in some of the children, lack of proper nourishment. Social Services provide assistance by means of a supporter at the home, as the mother does not function, even on the simple level of food and cleanliness. She behaves like one of her children, sitting and waiting for food to be served. She was not able to manage the kitchen and secure food in the refrigerator for the family, even when the supporter tried to help and teach her. The surrounding religious families help the family, but the crisis of chronic neglect is too severe to overcome.

The extended family (the parents) assist, but still this is a family with very low means of existence. Half the children attend special education due to learning difficulties and developmental delays. Partly this is due to environmental deprivation and lack of stimuli. All the children had normal pregnancy and delivery without any apparent genetic or hereditary deficiency. Most of the children attended the child development center, because of delay in motor and speech development, but some of them also displayed under- and malnourishment.

There is no doubt that this family, most specifically in regard to the mother since the father is hardly at home, is not capable of raising the children, especially such a large number. This family is not prepared to consider birth control, even with rabbinical intervention or suggestion.

The mother maintained that it is a religious command to have children and she is not interested in preventing further children, even if their rabbi said otherwise. She also resisted the placement of her nine-year-old son with a foster family son (due to an extreme physical, emotional and cognitive deprivation), and she is totally unaware of the suffering of her child. In general, the children are neglected, dressed unsuitably (winter clothes in summer and the opposite), with chronic hair lice, very scarce vocabulary and developmental delays. There was a wide gap between the ability of the mother to function, and her desire to rear her children at home, which is largely explained by her intellectual disability, where she is unable to understand the damage she is causing them. It was quite obvious that she evoked compassion from the community and professionals, including teachers, social workers and psychologists, due to the pressing needs of her children. The family social worker expressed frustration and a sense of helplessness, when she spoke of the future for these children and said over and over: "it is not fair towards the children."

DISCUSSION

Rabbi Samson Raphael Hirsch noted: "Concerning education for moral perfection, there is no substitute for the care given by the mother," and the Talmud states that the reward to women is greater than that to men, because the main responsibility for educating the child belongs to the mother (Matzner-Bekerman, 1984). The father has responsibility for certain aspects of the education of the child, but the mother has the responsibility for the child's primary spiritual and moral learning (Matzner-Bekerman, 1984). Teaching takes patience and skill, which can be seen from the following example from the Talmud (Eruvin 54b):

> Rabbi Preida had a student to whom he would have to repeat each lesson four hundred times before he understood it. One day (R. Preida) was required to leave and attend to a certain matter involving a mitzvah. Before leaving, he taught (the student) the usual four hundred times, but he still did not grasp the lesson. (R. Preida) asked him, "Why is today different?" (The student) answered him, "From the very moment they told master that there is a mitzvah matter for him to attend, my attention was diverted, because every moment I said that now the master will get up and leave: now the master will get up and leave." (R. Preida) said to him, "Pay attention and I will teach you." He taught him again (another) four hundred times. A Heavenly voice emanated and asked (R. Preida), "Do you prefer that four hundred years be added to your life, or that you and your generation merit the life of the World to come?" (R. Preida) replied: "That I and my generation merit the life of the World to come." The Holy One, blessed is He, said to them: "give him both this and this."

Rabbi Preida showed that dedication and individual attention are the necessary ingredients for a teacher to succeed with his students. This patience and ability should also be required of and granted to every parent.

In this paper we have discussed the attitude of Jewish Law toward the marriage of persons with intellectual disability and found that there is no prevention of such a marriage. They may even have children within the framework of the law. Nevertheless, we presented an anecdote with two parents with intellectual disability who were not able to provide basic needs for their children, and the dilemma of Social Services on how to provide a safety net for these children.

Jewish Law is more liberal than American Law in this regard. The Mental Deficiency Act of 1913, as an example, made marriage illegal for persons with mental retardation everywhere in the United States (Randolph, 2003). This has changed, and thus the future will therefore see many more cases, even though data is scarce today. It has been estimated (Randolph, 2003) that there are approximately 1.4 million parents with intellectual disability in the United States between the ages of 18-64 years with children under 18 years.

The main issue involved is the welfare of the children, both when we discuss children of parents with mental illness (Hetherington et al., 2002) or intellectual disability (Whitman & Accardo, 1990). Data from the United States, the United Kingdom and Australia (Randolph, 2003) is beginning to demonstrate that parents with intellectual disability are:

- overrepresented in child-care proceedings.
- less likely to have received support in their parenting.
- at greater risk to have their parental responsibility terminated on data that would never hold in a case of non-disabled parents.
- likely to have their competence as parents judged against stricter criteria or harsher standards than other parents.
- more likely to have their children removed and their parental rights terminated.
- disadvantaged in the child protection and court process by rules of evidence and procedure.
- less likely to receive support in correcting the conditions leading to termination.

These factors are reported even though we have little evidence that having parents with intellectual disability will have an adverse effect on the child. Our case was just a case of the adverse effects and there may be other cases, where other factors will influence events in a positive direction.

Researchers from Sheffield Department of Sociological Studies (Booth & Booth, 2000) studied 30 people (16 men, 14 women), aged 16-42 years of age, who had grown up in a family with one parent (28 cases) with intellectual disability (usually the mother, 25 cases), with follow-up in-depth interviews. Of the 30 people half were themselves with learning difficulties, which was more than expected. None of these 30 people had had an easy childhood; 11 admitted skipping school, 11 had been in trouble with the police (three served time in prison), two had attempted suicide, 11 were divorced, 16 had experienced some form of abuse, seven presented or had overcome mental illness, and eight suffered chronic illness. The overall findings showed that not all children were the victims of their situation and many demonstrated adaptability in coping with a life full of difficulties. There was not a direct correlation between parenting skills and child outcomes, since outcome depended on more that just the parents and it appeared that the support system had had a positive effect. The (now) adults displayed a close relationship with the parents (especially their mother), which was the heart of their adult identity.

CONCLUSIONS

Jewish Law has been very progressive in the possibility of marriage between persons with intellectual disability in contrast to American Law, where this right historically has been denied, because of the assumption that the children would be better off not being born or being taken care of by others.

In the case of such a union resulting in children, although they require some supervision, family, friends and social welfare agencies have scrutinized these families to the extent that the parents feel a constant fear of their child being taken away.

There is little information on the number of such cases, and an overall dearth of information regarding the effects on the children, although one recent study from the United Kingdom has shown a varied picture of resilience and a close warm relationship later on with their family and especially the mother.

REFERENCES

Booth, T., and Booth, W. (2000) Against all odds: Growing up with parents who have learning difficulties. *Mental Retardation 38*(1), 1-14.

Farbstein, M. (1995) *Legal principal and clarification of the daat concept and laws concerning the shotah.* Jerusalem: Shaar Hamispat Institute [Hebrew].

Hetherington, R., Baistow, K., Katz, I., Mesie, J., and Trowell, J. (2002) The welfare of children with mentally ill parents. *Learning from inter-country comparisons.* Chichester, UK: John Wiley.

Jakobovits, I. (1959) *Jewish medical ethics. A comparative and historical study of the Jewish religious attitude to medicine and its practice.* New York: Bloch.

Lifshitz, H., and Merrick, J. (2001) Jewish law and the definition of mental retardation: The status of people with intellectual disability within the Jewish Law in relation to the 1992 AAMR definition of mental retardation. *Journal of Religion, Disability & Health 5*(1), 39-51.

Matzner-Bekerman, S. (1984) *The Jewish child: Halakhic perspectives.* New York: KTAV.

Merrick, J., Gabbay, Y., and Lifshitz, H. (2001) Judaism and the person with intellectual disability. *Journal of Religion, Disability & Health* 5(2/3), 49-63.

Randolph, R. (2003) *Information packet: Parents with mental retardation and their parents*. New York: Hunter College, School Social Work.

Whitman, B., and Accardo, P. (1990) *When a parent is mentally retarded*. Baltimore: Paul H Brookes.

doi: 10.1300/J095v10n03_12

The Participation of Disabled Women in the Rules of *Niddah*

Deena R. Zimmerman, MD, MPH

SUMMARY. In Jewish Law (*Halachah*) a woman is in the state of *niddah* after uterine bleeding. This short paper explains the laws concerning *niddah* and also aspects involving the women with disability. doi:10.1300/J095v10n03_13 *[Article copies available for a fee from The Haworth Document Delivery Service: 1-800-HAWORTH. E-mail address: <docdelivery@ haworthpress.com> Website: <http://www.HaworthPress.com> © 2006 by The Haworth Press, Inc. All rights reserved.]*

KEYWORDS. Disability, women, Jewish law, *niddah*, Israel

One of the cornerstones of Jewish law (*halachah*) is the conduct of a woman who has the religious status of *niddah*. This status is brought on by uterine bleeding. The most common cause of this situation is menstruation, but it can also be caused by side effects of medications such as

Deena R. Zimmerman is a specialist in pediatrics with clinical work at the TEREM-Immediate Medical Services in Jerusalem and Macabi Health Services in Shaalvim and researcher at the National Institute of Child Health and Human Development, Saban Children's Medical Center, Soroka University Medical Center, Beer-Sheva, Israel (E-mail: yoatzothalacha@nishmat.net).

[Haworth co-indexing entry note]: "The Participation of Disabled Women in the Rules of *Niddah*." Zimmerman, Deena R. Co-published simultaneously in *Journal of Religion, Disability & Health* (The Haworth Pastoral Press, an imprint of The Haworth Press, Inc.) Vol. 10, No. 3/4, 2006, pp. 217-220; and: *Jewish Perspectives on Theology and the Human Experience of Disability* (ed: Rabbi Judith Z. Abrams, and William C. Gaventa) The Haworth Pastoral Press, an imprint of The Haworth Press, Inc., 2006, pp. 217-220. Single or multiple copies of this article are available for a fee from The Haworth Document Delivery Service [1-800-HAWORTH, 9:00 a.m. - 5:00 p.m. (EST). E-mail address: docdelivery@haworthpress.com].

hormonal contraception and midcycle bleeding. Childbirth brings on a similar status as well. Much has been written about the reasons for this practice. The focus of this article, however, is the inclusion of disabled women in this practice both in Talmudic times and at present.

THEORETICAL BACKGROUND

Niddah is a halachic status that women enter, when they experience uterine bleeding not due to abrasions, lacerations or other forms of trauma. While the most common cause of this status is menstruation, *niddah* and menstruation overlap, but are not totally synonymous. Uterine bleeding from the withdrawal of hormones (such as occurs when using oral contraceptive pills), and as side effects of medication also causes the onset of this status. Stains found on the body, clothing or bedding that fit certain criterion and cannot be attributed to other sources (known as *ketamim*), also render a woman *niddah*. Opening of the cervix beyond a certain minimum size, such as is sometimes done during gynecological procedures, renders a woman *niddah,* even in the absence of visible bleeding. Childbirth brings on a similar status known as *yoledet.*

A woman remains in this status until she passes a number of stages:

1. All bleeding has ceased as halachically confirmed by a self-performed internal exam known as a *hefsek taharah* and further confirmed by the insertion of a cloth in a procedure known as a *moch dachuk.* If the bleeding episode has been short, there is still a required minimum of five days (or four by some Sephardi customs), since the onset of the status.
2. Seven days have passed that start the day after the five days or *hefsek,* whichever is later. During these days, the woman performs internal exams known as *bedikot* (generally two per day) that halachically assure that bleeding has not restarted.
3. On the completion of the seven clean, white, or blood-free days (known as *shiva nekiim*), and after procedures done to assure that there are no foreign substances left on her body (known as *eeyun* and *chafifah*), the woman immerses in a kosher *mikveh* (ritual bath). She then resumes her halachic status of *tehorah.*

At the time when there was a temple in Jerusalem, a woman with this status was proscribed from preparing foodstuffs that required ritual purity. In the absence of the temple, this is currently not relevant. However, being *niddah* still has religious significance. While the wife is *niddah*, a couple is not permitted any physical contact. There are further proscriptions on behavior, known as *harkhakot*, that apply as well. In order to prevent inadvertent marital relations at the time that a woman commences her menses, the couple also observes times of separation (*vestot* or *onot perishah*) when marital relations, and according to some customs hugging and kissing as well, are prohibited, but the *harkhakot* are not required.

SOURCES OF INCLUSION OF DISABLED WOMEN

The mishna in the tractate *Niddah* states:

> [For] deaf, mentally incompetent (shoteh), blind and insane women, mentally competent women prepare them and then they can eat terumah [one of the foodstuffs that has to be eaten in a state of ritual purity]

The Babylonian Talmud (*Niddah* 13b) asks a number of questions about this *mishna*. The first question is: Why is the deaf woman included in this list? There does not seem to be any requirement for hearing in order to perform the preparatory actions outlined above. The Talmud answers that the mishna is referring to a deaf-mute. Due to the inability to communicate, a deaf mute is halachically considered legally incompetent. There is rabbinic debate as to the status of a deaf-mute, who can communicate via sign language, but discussion of this is beyond the scope of this article (see Steinberg, A., *Encyclopedia Hilchatit Refuit* [Heb.] Jerusalem: Machon Schlesinger, 1988). The Talmud then asks about the blind woman. Why cannot she do the exams herself and then just show the cloth to a woman with sight? In fact, according to Rabbi Yossi ben Rabbi Chaninah, the blind woman should not be part of this list. The next question is why it lists both an insane and a mentally incompetent women–are they not the same? The Talmud explains that the insane refers to a woman who has become incompetent based on illness, apparently in contradistinction to a woman who has been developmentally disabled from a young age, or perhaps a temporary condition as opposed to a permanent condition.

The relevance of this mishna and its Talmudic glosses to our thesis is to show the assumption that these women are part of the ritual and thus appropriate accommodations need to be made for them.

The *Shulchan Aruch* (*Yore Deah* 198:28), the central code of Jewish law, discusses immersion by women who need assistance to do so. It states that other women can hold them during immersion as long as they wet their hands previously (and thus there is no interruption between the woman immersing and the water of the *mikveh*). Numerous responsa show that this includes women, who are unable to stand, i.e., with physical disabilities.

Many modern *mikvaot* make arrangements for disabled access. This can range from ramps into the building, special changing rooms with wheelchair access and/or include lifts to get into the water. Organizations such as TODA (Torah Organization for Disability Access) in Israel can be helpful and Milbat (*www.milbat.org.il*), an organization for disability equipment, keep lists of such *mikvaot*. Even in the absence of such technology, other women will be found to carry a disabled woman into the *mikveh* to allow her to participate in this important ritual. At this moment it cannot be said that all *mikvaot* are disabled-friendly in Israel, but there is no question that it is an assumption within halacha, from Talmudic times on, that accommodations have to be made for the inclusion of the disabled in this part of religious practice. A personal experience is related by Chava Willig, disabled since adolescence due to polio, in her essay "A house of hopes" in Slonim, R., [ed] *Total Immersion* (Northvale, NJ: Jason Aronson, 1997).

doi: 10.1300/J095v10n03_13

Legal Aspects of Parenthood
Among Persons with Intellectual Disability
in Israel

Isack Kandel, MA, PhD
Katherine Bergwerk, MD
Joav Merrick, MD

SUMMARY. Persons with intellectual disability are living longer, more integrated into the community and participating more in normal behavior that includes marriage and parenthood. This can be seen as part of normalization and reflects a change in societal attitude towards people with intellectual disability. This paper examines different aspects of par-

Isack Kandel is Senior Lecturer at the Faculty of Social Sciences, Department of Behavioral Sciences, the Academic College of Judea and Samaria, Ariel. During the period 1985-93 he served as Director of the Division for Mental Retardation, Ministry of Social Affairs, Jerusalem, Israel (E-mail: kandelii@zahav.net.il).

Katherine Bergwerk formerly of the Cedars-Sinai Medical Center, Los Angeles, where she was Associate Clinical Professor of Ophthalmology, Jules Stein Eye Institute, UCLA, is now working in private practice in Israel (E-mail: Bergwerk@juno.com).

Joav Merrick, is Director of the National Institute of Child Health and Human Development, Division of Pediatrics, Faculty of Health Sciences, Ben Gurion University, Beer-Sheva and also Medical Director at the Division for Mental Retardation, Ministry of Social Affairs, Jerusalem, Israel (E-mail: jmerrick@internet-zahav.net).

[Haworth co-indexing entry note]: "Legal Aspects of Parenthood Among Persons with Intellectual Disability in Israel." Kandel, Isack, Katherine Bergwerk, and Joav Merrick. Co-published simultaneously in *Journal of Religion, Disability & Health* (The Haworth Pastoral Press, an imprint of The Haworth Press, Inc.) Vol. 10, No. 3/4, 2006, pp. 221-227; and: *Jewish Perspectives on Theology and the Human Experience of Disability* (ed: Rabbi Judith Z. Abrams and William C. Gaventa) The Haworth Pastoral Press, an imprint of The Haworth Press, Inc., 2006, pp. 221-227. Single or multiple copies of this article are available for a fee from The Haworth Document Delivery Service [1-800-HAWORTH, 9:00 a.m. - 5:00 p.m. (EST). E-mail address: docdelivery@haworthpress.com].

Available online at http://jrdh.haworthpress.com
doi:10.1300/J095v10n03_14

enthood in persons with intellectual disability, as seen through the eyes of the legal system in Israel today. doi:10.1300/J095v10n03_14 *[Article copies available for a fee from The Haworth Document Delivery Service: 1-800-HAWORTH. E-mail address: <docdelivery@haworthpress.com> Website: <http://www.HaworthPress.com> © 2006 by The Haworth Press, Inc. All rights reserved.]*

KEYWORDS. Intellectual disability, parenthood, legal aspects, Israel

Recent years have seen an increase in the number of people with intellectual disability (ID) living longer, moving to or already living in the community and also establishing relationships leading to marriage or to parenthood (Randolph, 2003). This is a part of normalization and a different societal attitude towards people with intellectual disability, but it also brings to focus different dilemmas and questions for the individual, the family, affiliated professionals and society. In this paper various questions concerning these dilemmas are posed and discussed from an Israeli legal perspective.

SHOULD A FEMALE WITH INTELLECTUAL DISABILITY BE "ALLOWED" TO BECOME PREGNANT?

There are no accurate and reliable figures on the number of parents with intellectual disability in Israel, which reflects the case worldwide. Several factors make this estimation difficult, such as fragmented services, poor records, lack of common definitions, missing assessments and the invisibility of many parents to official agencies. However, it seems that the number of parents known to practitioners is rising steadily. Most information about parents with an intellectual disability is derived from families, who are already known to the services, and therefore may be based on a skewed population, whose needs or problems are greater than those who are managing without formal support or intervention.

The question posed would maybe seem strange in the world today of normalization and de-institutionalization, because persons with intellectual disability are assumed to have equal rights. Nevertheless, it is a question that provokes the thoughts of many parents or professionals due to the grave responsibility of raising children produced by persons with ID and the question of their ability to care for their child(ren).

In Israel the 1962 Law of Legal Ability and Guardianship refers to all persons with intellectual disability, dependent individuals or anyone else who is unable to take full responsibility for his own affairs. In these cases the law rules that the court is permitted to appoint a guardian, who is either related to the individual, or any other person found fit for the role in the eyes of the court. The guardian then becomes responsible for this person and property.

In the United States, between 1900 and 1950, over 50,000 persons with intellectual disability were systematically sterilized (Kempton & Kahn, 1991) unknowingly or against their will (Braddock, 1998). This took place in 29 states, but over 50% of the cases were in California (Braddock, 1998). In the 1930s in Germany legislation resulted in forced sterilization of 300-400,000 persons, which culminated in the murder of about 250,000 persons with intellectual disability between the years 1939-1945 (Braddock, 1998).

Against the background of this history and the Holocaust, the attitude towards sterilization has been very strict in Israel. It is impossible for a residential care center for persons with intellectual disability to perform sterilization, but the guardian has the possibility to take the issue to court and ask the court for permission to have sterilization performed. In residential care centers for persons with intellectual disability in Israel, birth control measures are taken in order to prevent pregnancy.

The whole issue of sexuality in persons with intellectual disability has been a neglected area both in research and clinical practice (McCarthy, 2002). There has been very little research on how both women and men with intellectual disability experience and deal with their sexual lives. A few years ago the Division for Mental Retardation (DMR) in Israel established a course (one year duration) on sexuality for professionals working within the area of ID, and a center for consultation for persons with ID, their parents, care staff and professionals in order to deal with the taboo of sexuality in this population.

IN WHAT WAY IS IT POSSIBLE TO INTERVENE AND PREVENT CHILDREN FROM BEING BORN TO A COUPLE WITH INTELLECTUAL DISABILITY?

This aspect does not constitute a moral dilemma, when there is agreement on the part of the person with intellectual disability to terminate the pregnancy. On the other hand, if the female disagrees, the question arises if termination of pregnancy can be brought about by law.

In Israel up to 1977 abortions were performed on medical grounds. In 1977, the law was liberalized to include also family and social circumstances, but this aspect was deleted in 1979. Today a review of at least three persons (a physician with a specialty in obstetrics and gynecology, a physician with another specialty like family medicine, pediatrics, psychiatry or public health, and thirdly a social worker) can permit abortion under four situations: (1) to a woman under 17 or over 40 years, (2) pregnancy as a result of out of wedlock relationship, rape or incest, (3) suspected physical or mental disability of the fetus, and (4) danger to the physical or mental health of the mother (Kandel & Merrick, 2003). It is important to emphasize that the review committee can legalize abortion, but they cannot force an abortion. The person with intellectual disability, the guardian, or the courts are the only ones able to give the final permission to perform the abortion.

IN WHAT WAY IS IT POSSIBLE TO INTERVENE AND PROTECT CHILDREN BORN TO A COUPLE WITH INTELLECTUAL DISABILITY?

There is widespread belief that women with intellectual disability are unable to parent, which in many cases has resulted in termination of parental rights, but this topic continues to be very controversial (Parish, 2002; Randolph, 2003) and in need of further research.

The life circumstances of mothers with intellectual disability living in the community are often accompanied with many issues related to poverty, such as homelessness, insufficient monetary situation, insufficient nutrition, mental health problems, various sorts of abuse or neglect and medical problems (Parish, 2002). These factors can influence the mother-child interaction and bonding in negative ways (Osofsky & Fitzgerald, 2000; Iwaniec, 2004) and hamper child development, but one study did not find any significant difference between mothers with intellectual disability compared to mothers from similar socioeconomic backgrounds in decision-making or maternal knowledge (Tymchuk et al., 1990).

The greatest concern about mothers with intellectual disability is the issue of child abuse and neglect of their child. Research has not been able to find a higher prevalence of abuse and neglect in this population compared to similar socioeconomic groups, but neglect has been observed as a result of inadequate training, support and supervision (Tymchuk & Feldman, 1991). From this experience it seems that mothers with intellectual disability in the community can parent and get help in this role, if intervention is adequate, supportive and adapted to their cognitive status.

Most research on children of parents with intellectual disability has focused on children up to three years of age. There is scarce research on long-term follow-up of these children. Recently researchers from Sheffield Department of Sociological Studies (Booth & Booth, 2000) published a study on 30 people (16 men, 14 women), aged 16-42 years of age, who had grown up in a family with one parent (28 cases) with intellectually disability (usually the mother, in 25 cases) with follow-up and in-depth interviews. Of these 30 grown-up children, half were intellectual disabled and none seemed to have had an easy childhood. Eleven had skipped school, 11 had been in trouble with the police with three having served time in prison, two had attempted suicide, 11were divorced, 16 had experienced some form of abuse, seven presented or had overcome mental illness, and eight suffered chronic illness. In spite of these findings, many also demonstrated adaptability in coping with a life full of difficulties. There was not a direct correlation between parenting skills and child outcomes, since outcome depended on more than just the parents, and it appeared that the support system had had a positive effect.

In case of abuse or neglect, the Child Protection Service of the Ministry of Social Affairs in Israel can remove a child from his home to residential or foster care, but the final decision is a court decision.

In Israel a Law on Adoption was enacted in 1981 (Weiss, 2001), where it is possible to arrange for adoption of a child in two ways. The first option is when the biological parents voluntarily consent to the adoption. The second option is through the termination of parental rights by the court. There are eight grounds for the Court to terminate parental rights:

- There is no reasonable possibility to locate or identify the parents or determine their opinion
- Where the parent is the father of the child and not married to the mother, has not recognized the child as his own and has unreasonably refused to take the child into his home
- Where the parent has died or been declared a legal incompetent or has had his guardianship over the child annulled
- Where the parent has abandoned the child or has unreasonably failed to maintain personal contact with the child over a continuous period of six months

- Where the parent has unreasonably failed to fulfill his parental obligations to the child, totally or with regard to his principle obligations, for a continuous period of six months
- Where a child under six years of age has been raised outside the parental home for a period of six months and the parent has refused, without justification, to take him into his home
- Where the parent is incapable of properly caring for the child due to his conduct in the near future, despite reasonable economic aid and treatment as are usually provided by the welfare authorities for purposes of rehabilitation
- Where the parent's refusal to consent to the child's adoption stems from an immoral motive or illegal purpose.

Termination of parental rights petition may only be filed in Court by the Attorney General or his representative. Most cases (100-150 cases in Israel per year) are based on the ground of the parent being unable to care for the child and there is no chance to change the situation despite efforts by the welfare authorities to support and assist (Weiss, 2001).

CONCLUSION

The fear and concern about reproduction in persons with intellectual disability has changed over time, from the former active intervention of mass sterilization to more normalization. Little research has been conducted *concerning* parenting by persons with intellectual disability and there are very few studies of long-term follow-up of children born to such parents. A recent study from Sheffield with 30 children now aged 16-42 years showed that none had had an easy childhood and, in fact, half were themselves with intellectual disability. Further research is needed, especially how to intervene and find support that works.

REFERENCES

Booth, T., and Booth, W. (2000) Against all odds: Growing up with parents who have learning difficulties. *Mental Retardation 38*(1), 1-14.
Braddock, D. (1998) Mental retardation and developmental disabilities: Historical and contemporary perspectives. In: Braddock, D., Hemp, R., Parosh, S., & Westrich, J., Eds. *The state of the States in developmental disabilities*. Washington, DC: AAMR, 3-21.

Iwaniec, D. (2004) *Children who fail to thrive. A practice guide*. Chichester, UK: John Wiley.

Kandel, I., & Merrick, J. (2003) Late termination of pregnancy. Professional dilemmas. *Scientific World Journal* 3, 903-912.

Kempton, W., & Kahn, E. (1991) Sexuality and people with intellectual disabilities: A historical perspective. *Sexuality and Disability* 9(2), 93-111.

McCarthy, M. (2002) Sexuality. In: Walsh, P.N. & Heller, T., Eds. *Health of women with intellectual disabilities*. Osney Mead, Oxford: Blackwell Science, 90-102.

Osofsky, J.D. & Fitzgerald, H.E. (2000) *WAIMH handbook of infant mental health. Parenting and child care*. New York; John Wiley.

Parish, S.L. (2002) Parenting. In: Walsh, P.N. & Heller, T., Eds. *Health of women with intellectual disabilities*. Osney Mead, Oxford: Blackwell Science, 103-120.

Randolph, R. (2003) *Information packet: Parents with mental retardation and their children*. New York: Hunter College, School Social Work.

Tymchuk, A.J., Tokota, A., & Rahbar, B. (1990) Decision-making abilities of mothers with mental retardation. *Research in Developmental Disabilities*, 11, 97-108.

Tymchuk, A.J., & Feldman, M.A. (1991) Parents with mental retardation and their children. Review of research relevant to professional practice. *Canadian Psychology* 32, 486-494.

Weiss, E. (2001) *Adoption in Israel*. Jerusalem: Ministry of Social Affairs.

doi: 10.1300/J095v10n03_14

The Sages, People with Disabilities, and Adaptive Technology

Robert Brown

SUMMARY. Adapting religious traditions by using new methods and technologies to be more inclusive is not new. This article explores how the system of the Jewish sages made participation and inclusion within Judaism possible for constituents who were excluded by its predecessors–especially people with disabilities. doi:10.1300/J095v10n03_15 *[Article copies available for a fee from The Haworth Document Delivery Service: 1-800-HAWORTH. E-mail address: <docdelivery@haworthpress.com> Website: <http://www.HaworthPress.com> © 2006 by The Haworth Press, Inc. All rights reserved.]*

KEYWORDS. Sages, Judaism, inclusion, disability, adaptive technology

R. Shesheth was blind. Once all the people went out to see the king and R. Shesheth arose and went with them. A certain Sadducean

---

Robert Brown is a layperson with cerebral palsy with an interest in Judaic studies. He works full time at Carnegie Mellon University, and serves in a volunteer capacity at Kane Regional Center in Scott Township near Pittsburgh, PA. This article was written in conjunction with his work with Rabbi Abrams and *Maqom*.

Address correspondece to: Robert Brown, 111 West Steuben Street, Pittsburgh, PA 15205-2631 (E-mail: Rb2c@andrew.cmu.edu).

[Haworth co-indexing entry note]: "The Sages, People with Disabilities, and Adaptive Technology." Brown, Robert. Co-published simultaneously in *Journal of Religion, Disability & Health* (The Haworth Pastoral Press, an imprint of The Haworth Press, Inc.) Vol. 10, No. 3/4, 2006, pp. 229-241; and: *Jewish Perspectives on Theology and the Human Experience of Disability* (ed: Rabbi Judith Z. Abrams and William C. Gaventa) The Haworth Pastoral Press, an imprint of The Haworth Press, Inc., 2006, pp. 229-241. Single or multiple copies of this article are available for a fee from The Haworth Document Delivery Service [1-800-HAWORTH, 9:00 a.m. - 5:00 p.m. (EST). E-mail address: docdelivery@haworthpress.com].

came across him and said to him: The whole pitchers go to the river, but where do the broken ones go to?

THE TALMUD

To study [medicine] diligently is among the greatest acts of worship.[1]

–Maimonides

When Rabbi Abrams asked me to submit an article on Judaism as it relates to issues of disabilities and health, I was at once and at the same time pleased and hesitant to attempt it.

By way of introduction, by the time some of you may be reading what I have to say in this article, I will be fifty-six years of age. My disabling condition is congenital cerebral palsy; up until my fortieth birthday, my primary mobility aid was a pair of Canadian crutches. Due to an accident in 1988 in which I was severely injured while crossing a busy Pittsburgh street, my mobility these days is accomplished with the use of a lightweight Quickie brand wheelchair. I live in Pittsburgh, Pennsylvania, where I have been employed at Carnegie Mellon University for the past twenty-seven years doing data entry with the use of a computer. I have two grown daughters named Suzanne and Sarah. After the premature death of their Mother, Lois, the responsibility for their care and nurture was mine. I had good support from my in-laws, who encouraged me in my tasks and helped keep our family unit together and whole in many different ways.

I am the one of two children who were the product of a mixed marriage–a mother who was nominally Jewish, and a non-Jewish father who was not observant within any form of organized Christianity, as far as I know.

Most of what I know about the Jewish and Christian traditions I learned as an adult; nevertheless, I consider these two to be a very important part of my personal narrative. I have taught, or been a participant in Jewish, Christian, and interfaith settings. For the past three years, I have been an active participant and student of Rabbi Abrams through the Maqom Adult Talmud Study Project. Maqom is an Internet Web site moderated by Rabbi Judith Abrams that makes distance learning and discussion of the Babylonian Talmud a possibility to people who might otherwise find such a task too daunting to attempt by themselves, or who would not otherwise be able to make the physical effort to begin to find a teacher.

I was pleased that Rabbi Abrams thought me articulate and educated enough to undertake such an article, but I hesitated, not because I am disabled, but rather because there are people with a range of many different disabilities just as there are many different types of Judaism. As soon as one makes a statement that generalizes a specific disability or health issue, there is a real risk that someone will say that their disability or illness affects them entirely differently from anyone else with the same diagnosis. I would be the first to concur on this point.

I would also point out that it is generally more difficult for someone who has been able-bodied to become disabled (as a result of an accident, or an illness thrust upon them) and to suddenly have to come to terms with it and accept the new limitations it may impose on lifestyle in terms of physical or mental ability, diet, or forced changes in living arrangements, than it is for one whose disability or illness is congenital or acquired through a mishap in the process of delivery. Again, while I certainly make no claim to being an "expert" in either the former or the latter case, I do consider that I have experience in both of these situations.

How does any religious tradition help people to cope with illness or disability? Where does one start to look for the evidence? Perhaps one of the best places to start would be in the foundation texts themselves.

In Christianity, for example, the Gospels are replete with stories of miraculous healings of people with various physical or mental illnesses. These stories seem to make the first two thirds of the Bible, what Christians have commonly called "The Old Testament," pale by comparison because while there are indeed some miracles of healing recorded within the confines of these pages, there seem to be certainly not as many as in the Gospels. Of course, what probably has been forgotten by many Christians who read these stories today is the apocalyptic or "end of days" nature of the original Christian message. The stories that illustrate these miraculous healings and that God was with them and active in the day-to-day life of the early believer were regarded as proof by its early adherents of the truth of Christianity. God was about to make His Kingship of the world evident for all to see, and these miracles of healing were signs that this event was imminent.

Anyone who has read these stories also sees another underlying message within them. In the opinion of the gospel writers, the society which is mirrored in these stories is sick, and in need of healing. I believe the way healing is accomplished through miraculous means in these stories is a direct result of their foundation in apocalyptic thought.

SCENES FROM THE TALMUD OF INCLUDING PEOPLE WITH DISABILITIES

So what about the Jewish tradition? Is there something specific to the Jewish traditions that might help an individual better cope with illness or disabilities? Do the sages have a different definition of disability; do many of us miss the point in our conception of what wholeness is? I believe the answer to both questions is a definite "yes."

I believe the sages also saw a society that was in need of healing–indeed they were part of it–but their prescription for recovery was oriented differently and, at times, perhaps more radical.[2] They also read the Bible but there was nothing particularly dated or old about it as far as they were concerned. Rabbinic Judaism could also be considered to have a canon that consists of two parts, one of them was the Bible, and the other was the Talmud, which gave new meaning to the way things were done and who could participate.

One of the institutions that the sages held in common with early Christianity was the institution of discipleship. We read in the Talmud, "One who teaches another's child Torah is regarded by the tradition as one who gave birth to the child" (B. Sanhedrin 19b). Unlike its predecessor, Temple Judaism, which was based on lineage and caste, the system of the sages was based on *da'at,* or correct knowledge or practice. This innovative approach to Judaism made direct participation in the system accessible for many more people. It was a more dependable system simply because it was not based on either dynastic succession, as was kingship in earlier times, or lineage, as in the Temple priesthood.[3] Here are some of many examples from the Babylonian Talmud. They relate some incidents in the lives of the sages R. Shesheth and R. Joseph. Both sages were blind:

> R. Shesheth[4] was once sitting in the synagogue which "moved and settled" in Nehardea, when the Shechinah came. He did not go out, and the ministering angels came and threatened him. He turned to him and said: Sovereign of the Universe, if one is afflicted and one

is not afflicted, who gives way to whom? God thereupon said to them: Leave him. (B. Megilah 29a)[5]

And,

> Rab said: [If the host says to his guests] Take, the benediction has been said, take, the benediction has been said, he [the host] need not say the benediction [again]. If he said [between the benediction and the eating], Bring salt, bring relish, he must say the benediction [again]. R. Johanan, however, said that even if he said, Bring salt, bring relish, the benediction need not be repeated. If he said, Mix fodder for the oxen, mix fodder for the oxen, he must repeat the blessing; R. Shesheth, however, said that even if he said, Mix fodder for the oxen, he need not repeat; for Rab Judah said in the name of Rab: A man is forbidden to eat before he gives food to his beast, since it says: And I will give grass in thy fields for thy cattle, and then, thou shalt eat and be satisfied. (B. Barachoth 40a)

> R. Shesheth also held that the Shechinah is in all places, because [when desiring to pray] he used to say to his attendant: Set me facing any way except the east. And this was not because the Shechinah is not there, but because the Minim[6] prescribe turning to the east. (B. Baba Bathra 26a)

Or take, as another example, this statement by R. Joseph:

> Originally, I thought that if anyone would tell me that the halachah agrees with R. Judah, that a blind person is exempt from the precepts, I would make a banquet for the Rabbis, seeing that I am not obliged, yet fulfill them. Now, however, that I have heard R. Hanina's dictum that he who is commanded and fulfils [the command] is greater than he who fulfils it though not commanded; on the contrary, if anyone should tell me that the halachah does not agree with R. Judah, I would make a banquet for the Rabbis. (B. Kiddushin 31a)[7]

The examples cited above from the Bavli may surprise some of us in that they illustrate that participation in the system of the sages was indeed possible by some groups of people with disabilities. In these examples, both R. Shesheth and his contemporary R. Joseph are blind but they still are able to participate and contribute to the give and take of discussion and debate that became part of the printed page of the Talmud. This was possible because much of what later became the printed page was transmitted orally and learned and retained aurally.

As with any system, no matter how inclusive, there were groups of disabled that were excluded from the sages' system. Mental disabilities and disabilities that affected speech and hearing kept people from participating in the sages' system.[8] Although this system was not all-inclusive (no system is, even today), it was ahead of its time in the way it included people and its use of the available technology of the day.

IMPLICATIONS OF THE SAGES' PROGRAM: TRANSLATION AS FACILITATIVE TECHNOLOGY AND THE TORAH AS CONSTITUTION

"The available technology of the day." How so? If I may, I should like to propose a theory here about the very nature of the Judaism of the sages that allows for its inclusiveness. Possibly more than any other Judaism of the time, the Judaism of the sages became a literary undertaking that was confined mainly between the pages of the Tanach and the Talmuds,[9] giving it a portability that its predecessors lacked since the time of the portable sanctuary known as the Tabernacle in the Torah. This, and the fact that the sages learned how to keep *Am Israel* together as a group without *Eretz Israel*, would give them an advantage shared with only one other religion of the time, Christianity (which itself was originally a Jewish sect and roughly contemporary with the Judaism of the sages). Comparatively, the literary form that was the Judaism of the sages, continued with the advent of rabbinic Judaism, and is akin today to the "computer revolution" in its implications regarding inclusiveness of people with disabilities within the wider Jewish communities. But, you might say, books have been around for thousands of years! How can they be compared to the personal computers and the internet that is available today in regard to the impact made on society as a whole, and more specifically, the benefit derived for Jewish communities in particular. Further, how have either books or computers benefited people with disabilities in terms of technology? Actually, I believe Judaism has a longer history in the field of adaptive technology than what first might be apparent. To start with the first technological advance that was needed, I ask the reader to consider this passage from the Tanach:

And all the people gathered as one man in the open place before the Water Gate; and told Ezra the Scribe to bring the book of the Torah of Moses, which the Lord had commanded to Israel.

And Ezra the Priest brought the Torah before the congregation both of men and women, and all who could hear with understanding, on the first day of the seventh month.

And Ezra the Scribe stood upon a platform of wood, which they had made for the purpose; and beside him stood Mattithiah, and Shema, and Anaiah, and Uriah, and Hilkiah, and Maaseiah, on his right hand; and on his left hand, Pedaiah, and Mishael, and Malchiah, and Hashum, and Hashbadana, Zechariah, and Meshullam.

And Ezra opened the book in the sight of all the people; for he was above all the people; and when he opened it, all the people stood up; And Ezra blessed the Lord, the great God. And all the people answered, Amen, Amen, lifting up their hands; and they bowed their heads, and worshipped the Lord with their faces to the ground.

Also Jeshua, and Bani, and Sherebiah, Jamin, Akkub, Shabbethai, Hodijah, Maaseiah, Kelita, Azariah, Jozabad, Hanan, Pelaiah, and the Levites, helped the people to understand the Torah; while the people stood in their places. So they read in the book in the Torah of God clearly, and gave the interpretation, so that they understood the reading. (Neh. 8:1-8)[10]

Now, this passage is interesting for many reasons. Let us focus in on just two of them, keeping in mind what I have stated above regarding the use of technology. At first glance, it seems as if the people gathered to hear the *Torah* read aloud were capable of understanding the reading of it in its original language, as perhaps many of them indeed were. However, we learn further in this passage that there were also a substantial number of the people who needed help to understand what was being read to them in the original Hebrew. These had returned from the exile in Babylonia without a knowledge of Hebrew; they spoke the language current in Babylonia at the time, Aramaic, a Semitic language like Hebrew but different enough from Hebrew to pose a problematic language barrier. What was done was to have people who had a technical knowledge of both Aramaic and Hebrew explain the reading so that all might comprehend, no matter which language each individual listener understood. While this passage may be one of the earliest references to the activity of translators, later called *meturgemanim*, they continued to provide such help in rabbinic times.[11] It was the task of these translators not only to translate the text but also to make it comprehensible to the listeners. Early rabbinic sources refer to the public reading of the Targum[12] alongside the reading of the weekly portion of the Torah. According to tradition this practice originated with Ezra:

> What is the meaning of, And they read in the book, in the law of God, distinctly, and they gave the sense, so that they understood the reading? "They read in the book, in the law of God," refers to Scripture; "distinctly," to Targum; "and they gave the sense," to the division of sentences; "so that they understood the reading," to the accentuation; others say, to the masoroth.[13] (B. Nedarim 37b)

If this was the first instance of use of a translation to facilitate the understanding of a text that had become incomprehensible to Jews who had never learned to read and understand the Hebrew original, it certainly was not the last. The Hebrew Bible was eventually translated into Greek where it became accessible to the Western world.

What I have described here is a very early use of translation as technology to make a text in one language comprehensible to people who spoke another even though they considered themselves (and were considered) as part of the same people. This understanding of community, for the time, is uniquely Jewish. Why was this important? To answer, let us return to the passage in Nehemiah. *"Torah"* is a Hebrew word that can have many meanings. These meanings can occur simultaneously or be shared consecutively within a passage, or the meanings can vary between one passage of scripture and another. Many modern Christian translations of the Bible render the Hebrew word *torah* as "law" in English. It is more correctly rendered as "teaching," as some modern Jewish translations do. Still others leave it untranslated, which is probably preferable, because no one English word can define the concept in the totality of all its nuances.

One of the many meanings that *"torah"* can convey to English is "constitution," in the sense that the *Torah* is the actual document that establishes the people as a nation and institutes the government. It limits the power the government can exercise over the governed, whether that power be exercised through the tribal confederations of early Israel, or still later, under the experiment with monarchy. It also gives the governed certain rights that are guaranteed by God. Indeed, the critique of the Prophets could be seen as one that was measured against how well or how poorly the royals governed by the *Torah* as constitution, even if that constitution was not exactly in the final form as the one read aloud by Ezra to the assembled congregation in the passage under consideration from Nehemiah. The Bavli and the *Torah* of Nehemiah also change, much the same as the U.S. Constitution has evolved from the one ratified by the thirteen original states. What these documents all have in common is that they are inspired and informed by the contemporary understanding of scripture; in short, we are discussing living and continuing traditions rather than history. Translation, at least in the case of the Tanach and Bavli, was a necessary technology so that *all* the people could agree and consent to be governed by its terms.[14]

The problem that both the sages and later rabbinic Judaism faced can be seen as a question of how to establish a government that would govern a people who had been deprived of a homeland that would ordinarily establish national and cultural boundaries that were at least recognized, if not respected, by other cultures. Further, this government could not be imposed from above, but had to be voluntary, and informed by the people who were actually to be governed. The major cultures to be reckoned with were the Greek, and later, the Roman. As for Rome, it borrowed much of what it considered beneficial from Greece, and continued the pattern under Constantine.

What the sages did within the pages of the Bavli was to remove Jews from active consideration of political matters in an attempt to insure their survival in a world that was hostile to them. This affects the very orientation from which the Bavli speaks to us as Jews. While the sages were indeed interested in preserving Jewish self-government and autonomy, they projected political concerns into a future messianic age by addressing themselves to the character of the nation when that age would arrive.[15] However, the Bavli's overall orientation is focused on this world. It thus took a different route than its sibling, early Christianity, which originally emerged from apocalyptic Jewish sectarianism. Daniel Elazar sums up the final result of this process in his discussion of the nature of Jewish polity as it was transformed in the Bavli:

> What emerged was an aristocratic republicanism in which instead of a hereditary aristocracy, there was an aristocracy of the learned, open and accessible to *all*. This, indeed, was the great foundation of the sages' claim to authority. On the one hand, with the demise of the hereditary priesthood as a factor in Jewish public affairs, the

sages insisted that *all Jews*[16] truly become what the Torah commanded them to be, namely, a kingdom of priests and a holy nation, and that they do so by fulfilling what the sages claimed was the covenant obligation of learning, which would in turn internalize God's authority within each of them. The most learned would become the leaders of the people, able to express authoritatively God's will through constitutional interpretation of the covenant texts on the basis of the oral Torah.[17]

CONTEMPORARY APPLICATIONS

Technology still has a role to play that has remained largely undefined in the realm of religious studies and people with disabilities. Although *da'at* will always be a prerequisite for people wishing to participate actively in the study of Talmud, the discipline is becoming more inclusive as technology becomes available. This is indeed good news for the people born with disabilities or anyone who becomes disabled through the onset of disease or accident.

One such technology has been a real timesaver for this author. It is a product of Adobe Software who make the Acrobat Reader program. Called Adobe Reader 6.0, it allows a computer with the installation of an English version speech engine to actually read aloud documents that have been created and formatted by using this new technology. Would it not be wonderful to imagine that future versions of the Soncino Judaic Classics Library would be packaged by Davka employing this technology, making the basic Jewish texts available to sight impaired individuals? If this was to become a reality, it would be much more affordable than the alternative of committing such texts to Braille, or even putting such texts on audiotapes or compact disks. Ironically, it would recall the original method by which these texts were communicated—orally!

The problem of the actual typing of an article such as this one is already well on its way to solution. There are programs that will recognize speech, and type what is spoken by the author into a document. While such programs are relatively new, improvements are being made in successive versions.

With the advent of modern computer technologies, the synagogue is not the only place to go to study; the primary texts upon which rabbinic Judaism is based have become accessible to anyone wishing to know what they hold. The Tanach is available in more than one version, and a complete version of the Soncino edition of the Bavli with English trans-lation. Search capabilities and notes have been available from Davka Judaic Software since the early 1970s for anyone wishing to purchase them. These have two advantages: the texts in this form are generally easier for the user to search electronically, and in the case of the Soncino edition Talmud, the cost to purchase one has been reduced by around two thirds or more of what it would be in traditional printed media form. I have heard also that there is to be a Steinsaltz edition of the Talmud with similar features to be available soon on CD-ROM.

Couple this with the accessibility offered by the internet, making long-distance learning a reality with the teaching of Jewish subjects on line, and a very real possibility exists for a new renaissance in the dis-semination of Jewish knowledge and tradition. From a personal per-spective, I would say that all who were interested would gain, but perhaps individuals with disabilities would be the ones to benefit most, especially if mobility was an issue. Type "Judaism" into any internet search engine, and one is surprised at both the number of results and, upon further investigation, their quality.

When I wanted such knowledge, there were places to go where I found people who I consider to be first rate. The first, although no lon-ger available on a regular basis, was sponsored by the World Zionist Organization, and appeared on the internet under the acronym of J.U.I.C.E. (Jewish University in CyberspacE). I took two courses in Jewish history which covered the periods from the Bible up to the postmodern world and the establishment of the modern State of Israel. My teacher for these courses was Howard Zvi Adel Adelman, a profes-sor who had formerly taught classes at Boston College before making aliyah to Israel. He now lives in Jerusalem. The courses were free ex-cept for the cost of the texts used in the courses, which were available from Amazon.com. An individual could purchase the texts or, in some cases, borrow them by loan through either the library facilities at Carne-gie Mellon University, or at the Carnegie Free Library system here in Pittsburgh. In my opinion, no better courses could have been offered for any price. Unfortunately, due to present circumstances and unrest in Is-rael, the J.U.I.C.E. program has had its resources severely limited.

I had always planned to begin to learn Talmud but it was one of those things that I would do "some day." I had attempted once to start such a class that was being offered by the J.U.I.C.E., but after participating for a short while, I knew that most of my fellow students were beyond any level that I might soon achieve. I also knew that the Bavli was not a document that one could study by oneself. I had purchased some of the volumes of the Steinsaltz edition Talmud in English, but I found the task of study very difficult indeed.

On one of many trips to the local Barnes & Noble Bookstore, I saw a book by Rabbi Judith Abrams. On the book jacket I read the printed question "So, you've purchased the Steinsaltz Talmud, now what?" I had to admit, I really did not know. On a whim, I purchased another book that Rabbi Abrams had authored that I thought might be of help in studying the Steinsaltz edition volumes that I had purchased. It was then that I saw Rabbi Abrams had a Web site which I soon visited.

One could say, "I signed up, and the rest is history," but that would be missing much of the point. The Maqom Web site offers anyone the chance to learn Talmud, starting with the basics, and to discuss and exchange ideas about various aspects of it with real people through the use of a personal computer and an internet connection. I have also been able to do private study with Rabbi Abrams which resulted in a published paper in the Maqom Web magazine, an ongoing project of the Web site. What more is there to say? The sages would have regarded such use of technology as a true blessing–perhaps even as miraculous. I know I look forward to every exchange in the ongoing discussion.

NOTES

1. Front piece in *Illness and Health in the Jewish Tradition: Writings from the Bible to Today*, edited by David L. Freeman and Judith Z. Abrams (Philadelphia: The Jewish Publication Society, 1999).

2. See this author's article "Decoding the Bavli: A Case Study." The article can be found at *The Maqom Journal for Studies in Rabbinic Literature.*

3. See Rabbi Judith Abrams' *Judaism and Disability: Portraits in Ancient Texts from the Tanach to the Bavli* (Washington, D.C., 1998; Gallaudet University Press), pp. 123-197.

4. R. Shesheth was a blind sage who lived in Babylonia around the fourth century, C.E.

5. All quotations from the Babylonian Talmud (Bavli) are taken from the Soncino edition, published on CD ROM by Davka Judaic Software, Chicago, IL.

6. One outside the Judaism of the sages.

7. R. Hanina's position, unlike R. Judah's, is that one who is able to fulfill the command, even though blind as in R. Joseph's case, is obligated.

8. Op. Cit., Abrams, p. 152, ff. Whether one could participate was subject to whether the disabling condition changed.

9. These are the Hebrew Bible and the Yerushalami (Jerusalem Talmud) and the Bavli (Babylonian Talmud).

10. The English translation used here is by D. Mandel published by Davka Software, Chicago, IL, 2001. The paragraph divisions are my own.

11. *The Jewish Study Bible*, Adele Berlin and Marc Zvi Brettler (Ed.). (New York: Oxford University Press, 2004) p. 1835.

12. This is a translation of the Torah text into Aramaic.

13. This came to mean the traditional reading.

14. For an overall concept of this theory, see the work *Covenant and Polity in Biblical Israel* by Daniel Elazar (New Brunswick: Transaction Press, 1998).

15. Ibid., Elazar, pp. 374-377.

16. Italics are mine, not Elazar's.

17. Ibid, p. 376.

REFERENCES

Abrams, Judith, Freeman, D.L. (Ed.) (1999) *Illness and Health in the Jewish Tradition.* Philadelphia: The Jewish Publication Society.

Abrams, Judith (1998) *Judaism and Disability: Portrayals in Ancient Texts from the Tanach through the Bavli.* Washington, DC: Gallaudet University Press,

Berlin, Adele, and Brettler, Marc Zvi (Ed.) (2004) *The Jewish Study Bible.* New York: Oxford University Press.

Elazar, Daniel J. (1998) *Covenant and Polity in Biblical Israel: Biblical Foundations and Jewish Expressions.* New Brunswick: Transaction Publishers.

Soncino Talmud on CD ROM (Chicago: Davka Judaic Software, 2001).

doi: 10.1300/J095v10n03_15

Jacob Who Loves the Sabbath

Rabbi Bradley Shavit Artson, MA

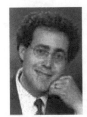

For ten years, I served as a congregational rabbi in the suburbs of Orange County, California, delivering many passionate sermons on the holiness of the Sabbath. I spoke of the need to reserve one day each week devoted to contemplation, to community, and to God. Quoting sources ancient and modern, I urged my congregants to abandon the headlong pursuit of elusive chores, of work never completed, and on this one day, to savor, instead, the simple wonder of being. But despite all those years of preaching Shabbat, and even though I myself was Sabbath-observant, I don't think I truly understood my own message or felt the full power of the seventh day until after I left the congregation. It was only after my fam-

Rabbi Bradley Shavit Artson is Dean of the Ziegler School of Rabbinic Studies at the University of Judaism, Bel Air, CA, and the author of *Dear Rabbi: Jewish Answers to Life's Questions* <http://www.nod.org/content.cfm?id = 1502>.

This article originally appeared in *Dancing on the Edge of the World: Jewish Stories of Love, Faith, and Inspiration* (2000), Miryam Grazer (Ed.), McGraw-Hill, pp. 63-66. Reprinted with permission.

[Haworth co-indexing entry note]: "Jacob Who Loves the Sabbath." Artson, Rabbi Bradley Shavit. Co-published simultaneously in *Journal of Religion, Disability & Health* (The Haworth Pastoral Press, an imprint of The Haworth Press, Inc.) Vol. 10, No. 3/4, 2006, pp. 243-246; and: *Jewish Perspectives on Theology and the Human Experience of Disability* (ed: Rabbi Judith Z. Abrams, and William C. Gaventa) The Haworth Pastoral Press, an imprint of The Haworth Press, Inc., 2006, pp. 243-246. Single or multiple copies of this article are available for a fee from The Haworth Document Delivery Service [1-800-HAWORTH, 9:00 a.m. - 5:00 p.m. (EST). E-mail address: docdelivery@haworthpress.com].

ily moved to the city that my six-year-old son Jacob showed me how to engage in the true soul-rest of the Sabbath.

Jacob gave me the gift of the Sabbath.

Jacob is autistic. His mind perceives the world in ways different from most people; his sense of timing and priorities follows its own inner schedule. The agendas that consume most of us simply don't exist for him. Jacob is indifferent to matters of social status. He loves what he loves, and he loves whom he loves. Jacob is passionate about his family, for example, cuddling in our bed early in the morning, sitting side-by-side as we read together, laughing as we chase one another around the park. And Jacob is passionate about the Torah; transforming a stray branch into a Torah scroll, he cradles it in his arms while he chants the synagogue melodies. Marching his "Torah" around the room, Jacob sings the ancient Psalms of David with the same joyous intensity of the ancient singer of Israel.

One of the insights–and challenges–of his autism is that unless Jacob loves it, it doesn't get his attention.

Once we moved into the city and I was freed from my obligation to arrive at services early, to stand on the pulpit, and to lead the congregation in prayer, I looked forward to savoring the early Shabbat morning walk to our new synagogue with my son. On our first Sabbath there, I tried to walk the way most other people walk. I wanted to arrive punctually. Jacob, on the other hand, was already where he wanted to be: enjoying a walk with his Abba. I cajoled, pulled, pushed, yelled, but Jacob would not rush. I told him we were going to miss the services, and still he strolled. I insisted that he hurry, and he paused to explore a patch of flowers, or sat himself down in the warm morning sun. I tried grabbing his hand and pulling him by force. I tried walking behind him and pushing with my knees. Nothing worked. By the time we arrived at the synagogue, hopelessly later, my stomach was in knots. I was drenched in sweat, and far too frustrated to pray.

The second week repeated the aggravation of the first. We still reached services late, and I was so annoyed that I couldn't even sit still when we did get to the sanctuary. This last week, I realized that something had to give. Jacob wasn't going to stop being Jacob, which meant that our walk would proceed his way, on his schedule. Resigned to slow frustration, I decided to make the best of it; I would learn to walk the way Jacob walked, but I would take a book.

I chose as companion a medieval mystical text by Rabbi Moshe Cordovero, the Tomer Devorah, "The Palm Tree of Deborah," a meditation on Kabbalah and Ethics.

As Jacob and I and Rabbi Cordovero set out on walk number three, I tried paying no attention to our speed or direction. When I got to the corner, I didn't let myself look at the light–invariably green until right before Jacob caught up. I read.

It's impossible to read quickly while you walk; reading while walking is a form of meditation: savoring individual words, delighting in phrases, I found the words on the page melding into my walk. "Who is like You, God?" the prophet Micah wrote. "There is no moment that people are not nourished and sustained by the Divine power bestowed upon them," responded Rabbi Cordovero. "Thus no persons ever sin against God without God, at that very moment, bestowing abundant vitality upon them. Even though they may use this very vitality to transgress, God is not withholding. Instead the Bountiful One suffers the insult and continues to enable the limbs to move." I could feel the vitality in the words infusing my own, making this very walk a celebration. The sunshine streamed into my soul, God bestowing life and love without conditions or restraint.

As I walked and read, the words of the Tomer Devorah reframed the morning song of a bird into an outpouring of creation's gratitude to God. The egglike flowers of the dogwood trees seemed to gesture the words of the psalmist, "How manifold are your works, O Lord. In wisdom you have made them all." In the towering palm trees we passed, I could feel the call of the prophet Isaiah, "Before you, mount and hill shall shout aloud, and all the trees of the field shall clap their hands."

From time to time, I turned around just to relish my son's meanderings. His joy was contagious: the pure delight of a little boy with his Abba and with time. And his joy was pure. My son cannot read, yet his very presence, I could now see, affirmed the words of the Kohelet that "there is nothing better than for one to rejoice in what he is doing." Occasionally, I found myself slipping into my old apprehensions, worrying about what part of the service I was missing, or fretting about not proceeding quickly enough. But the allure of my book, the walk, the sun, and my son, restored me. Jacob's spirit had become infectious.

When we finally did arrive at the synagogue, the service was more than halfway over. They were already putting the Torah scroll back into the Ark. Jacob squealed with delight, "The Torah! The Torah!" and ran to the front of the sanctuary. Too excited to stand still, he bounced on his toes next to the person holding the Scroll while the congregation recited the ancient praise: "Hodo al eretz v'shamayim! God's glory encompasses heaven and earth!" My spirit soared, for I had just borne witness to that glory in the flowers ablaze in color and light, in the delicate breeze swirling through the leaves. "God exalts and extols the faithful, the people Israel, who are close to God. Hallelujah!"

More than any sermon I've ever heard or given, I owe the fullness of the Shabbat to my son. Jacob taught me through his own example that we can't possibly be late, because, wherever we are, we are already where we are supposed to be. Our minds just have to acknowledge what our heart already knows.

I learned that day that Shabbat is the cultivated art of letting go, letting be, and letting in. In that art, my son Jacob is my teacher, my master, my Rebbe.

My Jacob gave me the gift of Shabbat.

BOOK REVIEWS

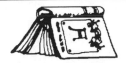

JUDAISM AND DISABILITY: PORTRAYALS IN ANCIENT TEXTS FROM THE TANACH THROUGH THE BAVLI. Abrams, Judith Z. Washington, DC: Gallaudet University Press, 1998, 236 pp., hardcover.

In this book you will find a review of the Jewish Bible–also called Tanach, the Mishna and the Talmud as it relates to disability. In the last chapter reference is also given to more recent Jewish scholars and their work (Mishneh Torah, Zohar, Arbaah Turim and Shulhan Aruch). The author of this book is a female rabbi and founder of Maqom, a school for adult Talmud study in Houston, Texas. The book was published a few years ago, but it is still relevant today and will be for years to come, as a classic study of disability in Judaism. The book is divided into seven chapters (Introduction; Priestly Perfection; Persons with Disabilities; Symbolism and Collective Israel; Disabilities, Atonement and Individuals; Body, Soul and Society; Categorization, Disabilities and Persons with Disabilities; and finally, The River Flows On). The focus to study the way disability affected Cohanim (priests) and their function in the Temple, how persons with disability were used as symbols of collective Israel, how individual life stories sometimes became literally object lessons in theology, how persons with disability were looked upon in Judaism and surrounding cultures, and how the person with disability was categorized.

[Haworth co-indexing entry note]: "Book Reviews." Co-published simultaneously in *Journal of Religion, Disability & Health* (The Haworth Pastoral Press, an imprint of The Haworth Press, Inc.) Vol. 10, No. 3/4, 2006, pp. 247-254; and: *Jewish Perspectives on Theology and the Human Experience of Disability* (ed: Rabbi Judith Z. Abrams, and William C. Gaventa) The Haworth Pastoral Press, an imprint of The Haworth Press, Inc., 2006, pp. 247-254. Single or multiple copies of this article are available for a fee from The Haworth Document Delivery Service [1-800-HAWORTH, 9:00 a.m. - 5:00 p.m. (EST). E-mail address: docdelivery@haworthpress.com]. Single or multiple copies of this article are available for a fee from The Haworth Document Delivery Service [1-800-HAWORTH, 9:00 a.m. - 5:00 p.m. (EST). E-mail address: docdelivery@haworthpress.com].

Available online at http://jrdh.haworthpress.com

One of the fundamental principles in understanding disability and Judaism is the term da'at (knowledge, understanding, intellect, cognition or consciousness). A person will have to have this in order to perform duties in Judaism; the person will have to be able to act upon his da'at and to put his da'at into action in the context of the society. The katan (the minor), the cheresh (the person with hearing and speaking disabilities) and the shoteh (the mentally ill, the intellectually disabled, the fool) are all in the same category of persons without da'at and therefore unable to perform a lot of duties in Judaism.

You will in this book find these terms defined, discussed and related in detail. Throughout the book you will find very illustrative comparisons to life today in order to explain sometimes difficult concepts for the modern person not engaged in religious life, like the comparison between the Marines and the Cohanim. Every American, at least, has heard the phrase "The Few, the Proud, the Marines" to give you a picture of the basic concept of able combat soldiers. When compared to the Cohanim, who also had to be an elite in a dangerous environment with many rituals and duties to perform in the Temple, it is easier to understand why there were restrictions on who could perform this Holy Duty and therefore perfection without disability. In this book, it comes out that Judaism and Jewish Law have had a very functional approach to disability and intellectual disability with a flexible view on the complex issues involved during a long history. I would recommend this book for scholars, for students and persons interested in Judaism. It is well-researched, with valuable notes and a good index. I was looking for some more information on the impact on modern Jewish life both in America but especially in Israel, after the establishment of a modern Jewish State, but I guess we have to wait for another book on that subject.

Joav Merrick, MD, DMSC
Professor of Child Health and Human Development
Medical Director, Division for Mental Retardation
Ministry of Social Affairs
Israel

DISABILITY IN JEWISH LAW. Marx, T. C. (2002). (Vol. 3 in the "Jewish Law in Context" series, edited by N. S. Hecht, Institute of Jewish Law, Boston University School of Law). London and New York: Routledge, 2002, xii + 260 pp.

Tzvi Marx has written a book of striking peculiarity. With an understanding yet critical "insider" eye he examines an enclosed world of rabbinical thought that concerns defect and disability, and that has been little concerned with presenting itself in an acceptable way to people outside the enclosure. Some of the contents would probably infuriate modern Western disability leaders (and also any feminists still interested in doing fury). Marx's aim is to expose, and suggest ways of reducing, some of the mutually contradictory interpretations within Jewish law (*halakha*) and the dissonance between Jewish law and modern Western secular beliefs and ideologies around disability.

The work had a prolonged gestation followed by a shadowy proto-existence, starting apparently in the late 1980s as Marx worked for his doctorate at Utrecht. The dissertation was accepted in 1993, and a few authors since then have cited the resultant weighty *Halakha and Handicap*.[1] The present book has a preface dated 1999, but almost all the references are from 1991 or earlier. Meanwhile, in 1998, Judith Abrams brought out her scholarly and well-written *Judaism and Disability*,[2] which innocently occupied much of the space on which Dr. Marx might have had first claim.

CLOSED AND INACCESSIBLE WORLDS?

The significance of the ten or twelve year gap is apparent throughout Marx's book. In the late 1980s, researchers even with some awareness of the nascent Disability Movement would still confidently produce crass generalisations, stereotyping "the disabled," their lives, their thoughts, the "problem and burden" they pose for family and society. So does Marx, e.g., "The disabled individual's simple physical dependency dominates family life" (p. 6); "The disabled are a population in chronic need of the generosity of others" (p. 69). In a publication of 2002, such

This review was first published in Disability World, No. 19, June-August, 2003. Reprinted with permission.

terminology and attitude sounds seriously dated. Still more incongruous is the use of "deaf-mute," in phrases such as "the closed and inaccessible nature of the deaf-mute's world until quite recently" (p. 114), on the same page as reference to "the hearing disabled." It is reasonable to use "deaf-mute" when discussing historical situations where that term was commonplace and not deemed offensive; but this exception hardly extends to phrases (and their implied thoughts) such as "deaf-mutes are today routinely taught to communicate vocally" (p. 234). Marx knows that terminology can be problematical, especially "the old associations with mental deficiency that the term 'deaf-mute' connotes in the halakhic mind" (p. 127). The problem is more in the "closed and inaccessible nature" of the world of halakhic debate, than in anything experienced by deaf or hearing-impaired people in the 20th and 21st centuries. Tzvi Marx has opened windows on an obscure and little understood world.

To understand what Marx has attempted, one must know that the world of traditional Jewish law does move, but very slowly because its roots are over two thousand years deep. For example, in 1988 when Jacob Neusner produced a fresh translation of the *Mishnah* (a foundational codification of Jewish law), deliberately using archaic English that adheres closely to the shape and order of the Hebrew text, he remarked that "the Mishnah is separated from us by the whole of western history, philosophy and science" (p. xxxiv).[3] This is the chasm that Marx faced, first in trying to understand and expound the authentic and dialectical teaching of earlier rabbis on disability, and secondly to bring out some underlying ethical principles. The latter give grounds from which the former may partly be refurbished, and this provides much of the interest of the book. Marx notes the need for skill to "navigate the intricate byways of halakhic logic" so that in any updating, if possible, "the empirical facts strengthen rather than undermine" what has gone before (p. 237). Each of the world's great religions and philosophies needs to undergo some refurbishment of its traditions and practices regarding disability and disabled people, and each naturally hopes to do so without admitting any abrupt contradiction of its earlier "authoritative" teaching.

Most religions and philosophies have embraced and taught some elevated charitable ideals, and these are prominently presented in Marx's exposition of Judaism with regard to disabled people. No doubt, for the great majority of humankind, balancing on the slenderest margin between survival and death, it has been good that the wealthy and powerful were exhorted to take thought for the poor and weak. However, in post-modern thought, balancing on an ample diet and a comfortable computer workstation, "charity" has become almost a dirty word, as Marx partly recognises when he notes that, "Charity, an offering of relief, is primarily remedial" (p. 69). The game now is to redesign the social environment so that having mental or bodily impairments, while still no doubt being a damned nuisance, should not dis-able anyone from living a fairly satisfactory life. Such a redesign might remove many of the occasions for high-minded "charitable practice," a removal for which erstwhile recipients would be extremely grateful (so the theory runs). Certainly, none of the great religions or philosophies can claim to be very far forward in the required reconstruction, refurb, or redesign.[4]

SEEKING DIGNITY AND MERIT

The traditional teaching and belief is that Jewish men seriously practising their religion are placed under 613 divine commands. These are not to be regarded as difficult, burdensome or constricting, but as a privilege and moral challenge from the creator (Marx, pp. 13, 28). There are differing views on whether the commands are all pragmatically good, i.e., embodying "The Manufacturer's Instructions" on how best to live life, or whether they are intrinsically good because they emanate from God, regardless of whether fallible humans can perceive in them any logic or reasonableness.[5] Either way, dignity is conferred on men by the effort to obey the commands and to order their lives by them. By contrast, the cow in the field is not (so far as we know) subject to commands–it faces no moral choice to be a good cow or a bad cow–whereas the religiously observant Jew acquires dignity by being commanded to keep every part of the law and making efforts to do so. One consequence is that those who were traditionally perceived as having a lesser obligation to keep the law, i.e., women, minors, and disabled people, seem inherently to have less dignity and less opportunity to acquire it. They may voluntarily try to keep some or all of the commands and this may count in their favour, or (as some rabbis have taught) perhaps such voluntary actions are a mistaken encroachment on territory that is inappropriate for them.

The previous paragraph gives (probably with foolish over-simplification) the gist of Marx's chapter 2, "Moral imperatives governing disability," in which he sets out the ground across which a modest number of Jewish teachers battled down the centuries, as elaborated in subsequent chapters. Considering every known or imagined flaw, impairment, difficulty or disability in the context of every one of the 613 legal dos and don'ts, the scholars have had plenty of tortuous material on which to disagree with each other and to cite reason, logic, linguistic gymnastics, ancient precedent and (sometimes) practical experience. In one location, some disabled people could be excluded from some activities either by legal purists ("they can't do it") or by the kind-hearted ("they need not do it"), with the risk of diminished human value. In another location, some could be included in the same activities either by legal purists ("they are not exempt") or by the fair-minded ("to exclude them would be a contempt"), or perhaps by the pragmatic ("let's not be stupid about this thing"). As a longstanding example, Marx points out that "the range of opinion on the halakhic inclusion of the blind in observance of the precepts varies from complete exemption, in Rabbi Judah's view, to almost total obligation . . . in Rabbi Meir's view" (pp. 106-107).

Contradictions within the major text-based religions over what is the authentic law, what is its meaning, and how it is to be applied in life-situations involving very different cultures and technologies, tend to reflect badly either on the wisdom of God or on the idea that God ever did "send down" well-drafted and universally applicable laws, beyond the very simplest and broadest principles for amicable co-existence ("don't eat other people"; "don't bother your father when he's watching the big game"). Some theologians of various religions have given up defending "revealed universal law" positions, and instead suggest a combination of progressive discovery and revelation: humankind collectively gropes toward practical ways of regulating community life and society so that the strong do not excessively oppress the weak, and the majority leaves some valued space for minorities, assisted and enlightened by nudges and hints from a deity who got bored with cows and thought up some creatures with capacity to evolve a mature moral sensibility (even if it takes several millennia). Tzvi Marx does not propound any such hypothesis; but the long centuries of slow and painful rabbinical debate tend to support the notion that life's rougher sides provide opportunities for moral growth, however reluctantly we may embrace them.

PRELIMINARY TREATMENT

To expect Marx to survey views much beyond the halakhic world might be excessive. His chapter on "extra-halakhic sources" does inspect some biblical and rabbinical material not strictly concerned with law; yet some of the exposition is curiously limited, e.g., the case of

King David on pp. 53-54. Marx gives a simplistic treatment of the text (II Samuel 5: 8), quoting Jewish commentators who suggest that David "had an instinctive, inborn revulsion for the lame and the blind, precisely as the text states," with a footnote that some discount the "plain meaning of the text." This "plain meaning" is then seen as illustrating what Marx believes to be a "virtually universal phenomenon of the disabled arousing primordial abhorrence," and on this assumption David's "achievement in overcoming it"–i.e., his kindness to the lame Mephibosheth [Meriba`al]–"is particularly admirable." It would be better to concede that the meaning of this brief passage is notoriously far from "plain." It has attracted a substantial literature, among which the Biblical scholarship was reviewed recently by Anthony Ceresko,[6] while Elena Cassin earlier placed it in detailed historical and linguistic context.[7]

After an arduous labour of many years, Marx claims only that his book is a "preliminary treatment that will encourage dialogue and further study" (p. xi), and his concluding chapter modestly aims to "assess strategies for mitigating the dissonance" between the more humane and the more legalistic sides of halakhic discourse on disability. If the present review makes a few criticisms, they should be understood in the same non-dogmatic spirit. Marx has taken pains to make an even-handed presentation of sharply differing halakhic points of view. Even where it becomes evident that he disagrees with some of them, he eschews adversarial positions that would merely provoke abreaction. He has made a major contribution to the slowly growing scholarship linking ancient and modern beliefs, attitudes and practices.

M. Miles
West Midland, UK

NOTES

1. Marx, T. (1993) *Halakha and Handicap: Jewish Law and Ethics on Disability.* Jerusalem: T.Marx (The British Library catalogue lists a copy of this, but the library had already mislaid or lost it by the time I made requests for it in the late 1990s. . .)

2. Abrams, J. (1998) *Judaism and Disability. Portrayals in Ancient Texts from the Tanach through the Bavli.* Washington DC: Gallaudet University Press.

3. *The Mishnah. A new translation* (1988) transl. J. Neusner. New Haven: Yale UP. The Mishnah, a somewhat idealistic compilation of Jewish oral law and interpretation reaching final form by the 3rd century CE, was the basis for further interpretative com-

mentary over a further three centuries, known collectively as the Talmud. Halakhic codification and interpretation has continued ever since.

4. Miles, M. (2002) Disability and religion in Middle Eastern, South Asian and East Asian histories: Annotated bibliography of selected material in English and French. *Journal of Religion, Disability & Health* 6 (2/3), pp. 149-204.

5. Cf. Abrams, *Judaism and Disability*, 152, who brings a new and improbable dimension to theological sources by her comparison of the Mishnah with the *Star Fleet Technical Manual* (based on the *Star Trek* TV series), since each contains some material dealing with theoretical situations unlikely to be met in real life.

6. Ceresko, A.R. (2001) The identity of "the blind and the lame" (`iwwer upisseah) in 2 Samuel 5: 8b. *Catholic Biblical Quarterly* 63: 23-30.

7. Cassin, E. (1987) *Le semblable et le différent. Symbolismes du pouvoir dans le proche-orient ancien*. Paris: Editions la Découverte. Two chapters discuss "Le droit et le tordu." The first (pp. 50-71) concerns disability in the Jewish scriptures, focusing largely on David, Meriba`al, and "the blind and the lame."

Resource Collections

Two Resource Directories from the United States for further Information:

1. *North American Disabilities Resource Directory of Jewish Agencies.*

Individuals, parents and professionals seeking information about programs and services in Jewish communities throughout the USA and Canada for children and adults who have disabling conditions now have a handy resource directory. The third edition of the *North American Disabilities Resource Directory of Jewish Agencies* has been published by The Council For Jews With Special Needs. The directory lists agencies, schools, camps, community centers, residential and vocational programs and other Jewish organizations that provide programs and services to children and adults who have developmental, physical, sensory, emotional and learning disabilities. The directory is arranged alphabetically by state and province. Copies of the directory in spiral bound hard-copy or on CD-Rom may be purchased for $30 (plus postage and handling) by contacting the Council at 480-629-5343 or by returning our ORDER FORM available at: *www.cjsn.org* (Resources).

2. *Dimensions of Faith and Congregational Supports for Persons with Developmental Disabilities and Their Families: A Bibliography and Resource Listing for Clergy, Laypersons, Families, and Service Providers.* 2005 Edition.

This 180-page resource guide has a six-page section on Jewish resources, including books, articles, agencies, videos and more. *Dimensions of Faith* is available in hard copy from The Boggs Center, P.O. Box 2688, New Brunswick, N.J. 08903 for $15 (shipping included). It is also available on the web, in PDF format, at: http://rwjms.umdnj.edu/boggscenter/products/prod_info.htm#dimensions

[Haworth co-indexing entry note]: "Resource Collection." Co-published simultaneously in *Journal of Religion, Disability & Health* (The Haworth Pastoral Press, an imprint of The Haworth Press, Inc.) Vol. 10, No. 3/4, 2006, p. 255; and Jewish Perspectives on Theology and the Human Experience of Disability (ed: Rabbi Judith Z. Abrams, and William C. Gaventa) The Haworth Pastoral Press, an imprint of The Haworth Press, Inc., 2006, p. 255. Single or multiple copies of this article are available for a fee from The Haworth Document Delivery Service [1-800-HAWORTH, 9:00 a.m. - 5:00 p.m. (EST). E-mail address: docdelivery@haworthpress.com].

Index

Abortion, 141n,223-224
Abraham, 115
Abuse
  by parents with intellectual
    disability, 224
  sexual, 141*n*
Accessibility. *see* Handicapped
  accessibility
Accommodations. *see also*
    Handicapped accessibility
  accessiblity training and, 165
  Community Inclusion Office's role
    and, 176-179
  family's role and, 179-181
  inclusion and, 158
  Minneapolis Jewish Federation and,
    171-173
  Niddah and, 220
  organizational roles and, 173-175
  physical barriers to, 166
  role of leaders for inclusion and,
    168-171
  schools' roles and, 176
  stumbling block principle and,
    136-137
  synagogues' roles and, 175-176
  Talmud on, 17
  for those with diabilities, 15-16
Adam, lonliness and, 13
Adaptive technology. *see* Technology
Adult care. *see* Residential programs
Age considerations, marriage and, 209
Aliyah, blindness and. *see* Blindness
Anemia, 152*t*. *see also* Genetic testing
Aristotle
  deafness and, 89,90-92
  infanticide and, 24*n*
Ashkenazic Jews

community presentations on Jewish
    genetic diseases and, 149-150
  conclusions, 152-153
  distribution of educational materials
    and, 149
  educational/screening event and,
    150-152
  introduction to, 148-149
  summary, 147
Attitudes, negative, 167
Autism, 243-246
Autonomy, 106
Avihu, 75-76

Bible
  Braille copies of, 15
  on exploitation, 17
  *Judaism and Disability: Portrayals
    in Ancient Texts from the
    Tanach through the Bavli,*
    247-248
  large-print copies of, 15
  loneliness and, 13
  marriage ceremony and, 208-209
  mitzvot and. *see* Mitzvot
Blindness
  aliyah/chanting the Torah and,
    34,42,44,46-47,51*n*
  commandments and, 72*n*
  conclusions, 47-48
  early modern practice and, 39-43
  Halakhah and. *see Halakhah*
  introduction to, 28-29
  Jacob and, 14
  as metaphor, 84
  obligation to keep mitzvot and,
    29-32

Cystic Fibrosis, 148,152t. *see also*
   Genetic testing

Daat kpeutot. *see* Marriage
Deafness
   accommodations and, 16
   ancient Judiasm and, 87-89
   Disability in Jewish Law, 250
   Greco-Roman history and, 86-87
   intelligence and, 89-94
   Judaism's teachings on, 14
   Mishnah and, 2,85-95
   sign language and, 97n
Death, obligation and, 24n
Decrees, rabbinic, overview of, 10
Dignity, *Disability in Jewish Law*,
   251-252
*Dimensions of Faith and
   Congregational Supports for
   Persons with Developmental
   Disabilities and Their
   Families,* 255
Disability. *see also specific disease
   names*
   a contemplation on, 5-8
   *Dimensions of Faith and
   Congregational Supports for
   Persons with Developmental
   Disabilities and Their
   Families,* 255
   Disability in Jewish Law, 249-254
   human rights and. *see* Human
     rights, disability and
   as individuated need, 143n
   intellectual. *see* Intellectual
     disability (ID), marriage and
   *Judaism and Disability: Portrayals
   in Ancient Texts from the
   Tanach through the Bavli,*
   247-248
   learning disabilities and. *see*
     Learning disabilities
   misconceptions regarding. *see*
     Misconceptions, disability

Niddah and. *see Niddah*
*North American Disabilities
   Resource Directory of Jewish
   Agencies*, 255
parenthood and. *see* Parents with
   intellectual disability
priests and. *see* Priests,
   requirements for
sterility and, 13
Talmud and. *see* Talmud
technology and. *see* Technology
theological considerations
   regarding. *see* Theological
   considerations
Disability in Jewish Law, 249-254
Discrimination. *see also* Inclusion
   discouraging, 169-170,173
   Judaism's teachings on, 14
Divorce
   get and, 64n
   grounds for, 65n
   incapacitated spouse and, 2,57-63
   remarriage and, 63n
   witnessing, 71n

Eastern European Jews. *see*
   Ashkenazic Jews
Economic considerations
   inclusion and, 158,170
   Jewish service providers and, 200
Eden, 120,142n
Education
   of others regarding disabilities, 163
   for special needs students,
     17-19,21-22
Embodiment, 6-7,12
Emotional conflict, Jewish service
   providers and, 200-201
Empathy
   inclusion and, 19-20
   Moses and, 22
Enactments, rabbinic, overview of, 10
Euthanasia, 55,118,141n
Eve, lonliness and, 13